I0410566

Body and Mind: NATURAL HEALTHY BALANCE

Dr. Elvis Ali, ND

Copyright © 2016 Dr. Elvis Ali

All rights reserved.

ISBN: 1539148270
ISBN-13: 978-1539148272

DISCLAIMER

The information in this book at all times is restricted to education, teaching and training on the subject of natural health matters intended for general natural health wellbeing and do not involve the diagnosing, prognosticating, treatment, or prescribing of remedies for the treatment of any disease, or any licensed or controlled act which may constitute the practice of medicine.

Questions? Please email us at: drelvisali10@hotmail.com

CONTENTS

ACKNOWLEDGMENTS

It is a pleasure to acknowledge with thanks:

My entire family in Canada and Trinidad and Tobago who have continued to support and motivate me to educate others about naturopathic medicine. My parents, Hakim, Hazrah, my sisters, Alima, Homaida, Homeeda, Fazida, my children, Hassan, Azeeda, Kareem, nephews, nieces and precious grandchildren, Gursimran, Meheirveer and Shairveer for their encouragement and belief in holistic medicine.

Colleagues in the healthcare profession, especially Dr. Leo Roy.

My students and staff at CCNM, BINM, CCHH, OAND, CAND and clinics, BTNL, AA Comfort Health Centers and Mississauga clinic. The companies for their assistance in educating the public about preventative medicine, Biorrific, Ecoideas, Canadian Bio, Sangsters, Fion Beauty Supplies Canada, Alpha Science Laboratories – A division of Omega Alpha Pharmaceuticals Inc.

My dear friends, Bonita, Pat, Roy, Cindy and Darryl, Janak, Joan, Ash and Harry, Saira and Moe Sheikh of Etobicoke Motors, along with many others too numerous to list.

My publisher and editor Sherree and Lillian who designed the book cover.

INTRODUCTION

Of course you want and expect that the treatments, recommendations and supplements you have received will succeed in restoring your health back to a level where you can live the life you want to live. What would be the point in following treatments if they didn't work?

But the point is that they don't and won't work unless they are used properly. This means...

- They constantly provide your body with everything it needs and all your body's cells need.
- That they are taken in the exact nature and proportion that they are needed.
- That you constantly refrain from, avoid and eliminate anything and everything that could be detrimental to your healing.
- All these needs must be constantly in balance – no less than your healing needs require – but also no more either.
- Every day your body's needs and balance change.
- You continue to persevere with your full treatment until your health is completely restored.
- *You* do all this.

You have to do all this! You have to do it without having done it before, without the training and experience to know how to do it perfectly!

Possibly you believe, like most people, that all you have to do is take the pills (supplements), make some changes in diet, and possibly make a few other prescribed changes and your treatment will automatically work.

Such an approach usually works for minor illnesses or

when treating only individual, simple symptoms. However, not if you are trying to correct a complex, multiple cause-type serious diseases.

If you have never built a house before, you would not attempt to do it on your own without help and guidance, and know-how.

The following pages will offer you some of these. They could mean the difference between a perfectly worked out healing program working for you - or not.

Understanding and appreciating your body, its organs and the way they interrelate and function as a team, is fascinating, morale building and encouraging. Self-knowledge creates a positive state of mind. It is a great step towards being you on a high level of wellbeing.

Bodies, minds and emotions – people are infinitely complex. Bodies are made up of hundreds of thousands of different chemical substances in their trillions of cells. Their minds, emotions and attitudes are just as complex. All these must be brought into harmony with the nature of the type of person you are and the nature of the life you lead. If not, many diseases remain incurable.

Healing and healing forces are not some abstract, nebulous mystery. They are the sum total and interacting team of...

- Morale, attitudes and emotions
- Support and influence of others around you
- The sum total of needed nutrients
- The biochemical and structural balances of all organs
- A lifestyle free of stresses, distress excesses and overloads.

Healing is done by very clear simple powers that are a normal part of our natures.

As one of the first full-time graduates from the Ontario College of Naturopathic Medicine (OCNM) now called (CCNM), we were taught to follow the six fundamental healing principles:

First: Do No Harm - Primum Non Nocere

Naturopathic medicine follows three principles to avoid harming a patient:

1. Utilize methods and medicinal substances that minimize the risk of harmful side effects.

2. Avoid, when possible, the harmful suppression of symptoms.

3. Acknowledge and respect the individual's healing process, using the least force necessary to diagnose and treat illness.

Your naturopathic doctor chooses remedies and therapies that are safe and effective, to increase your health and decrease harmful side effects.

Second: The Healing Power of Nature - Vis Medicatrix Naturae

Your naturopathic doctor works to restore and support the powerful and inherent healing ability of your body, mind and spirit, and to prevent further disease from occurring. Naturopathic doctors identify and remove obstacles to recovery, facilitating and augmenting this order and intelligent healing ability.

Third: Identify and Treat the Cause - Tolle Causam

The primary goal of your naturopathic doctor is to determine and treat the underlying cause rather than simply managing or suppressing the symptoms. The underlying cause may be due to diet, lifestyle habits, life events, posture or environment. Symptoms are viewed as expressions of the body's natural attempt to heal.

Fourth: Treat the Whole Person

Each person is unique and requires individualized care. In treating the cause of any condition, your naturopathic doctor takes into account not only your physical symptoms, but also mental, emotional, genetic, environmental, social, spiritual and other factors. Disease affects the entire person, not just a specific organ or system. Your nutritional status, lifestyle, family history, feelings, environmental stresses and physical health are all carefully evaluated, and addressed.

Fifth: Doctor as Teacher – Docere

Your naturopathic doctor will assist you in understanding health and illness. He/she will provide with an understanding of the factors that affect your health and help you balance, and become more capable of maintaining your own health. Naturopathic doctors also acknowledge the therapeutic value inherent in the doctor-patient relationship.

Sixth: Disease Prevention and Health Promotion

Your naturopathic doctor applies all of the above principles in a proactive form of disease prevention and health promotion. Naturopathic doctors emphasize healthy daily habits; they assess risk factors and hereditary susceptibility to disease and make appropriate interventions to prevent illness. Health is more than just the absence of disease. Health entails daily functioning on the highest possible levels and is obtained by proper nutrition, exercise, a balanced lifestyle, positive emotions, thoughts, and actions. The capacity for optimal wellness, or an improved quality of life, is inherent in every body.

Before starting treatments, and even while you are following them, read these pages. They are a part of your healing. Fix these concepts clearly in your mind. **Reread them periodically.**

- *YOU* are as much a part of your healing success as is your physician or counselor.
- *YOU* are responsible for all that is involved in your healing.
- *YOU* must know and avoid causes. Avoiding what causes disease is as important as taking remedies.
- *YOU* have to know and understand what heals and how healing works in order to heal properly.
- *YOU* can accomplish healing only with guidance by one who has learned to know the total you and your healing needs.

Learn them. Follow them. Neglect them at your own risk.

PART I

BODY HEALING

"A peaceful mind physically refreshes the body with both healing energies and a blanket of immunity." - J.J. Goldwag

1

False Cures

"Curing" is not aspirins, vitamins and drugs.

The "take-an-aspirin, cure-a-headache" way of thinking most of us have been conditioned to take for granted, leads us to believe that all cures work in simple ways. Such an approach may alleviate pain, infections and simple symptoms, sometimes even simple illnesses, but it does not heal any serious, ongoing, degenerative and life-threatening disease. It is like playing Russian roulette.

All substances that are not alive food from concentrates are drugs. Drugs work temporarily, but they do not a cure. They stimulate (whip) body functions and create rapid body changes, which may feel like healing. Drugs are appeasing, disease-perpetuating poisons that create smokescreens to a body's real needs and unrealistic expectancies. The only remedies that cure are those that supply every body's cell, mind and emotional needs, and correct every cause and influence, which created the disease abnormalities in the first place.

Healing Serious Diseases

Serious diseases are a serious matter. It is not to be approached lightly, dabbled with – try this, try that – shop from one doctor to another. There are no quick fixes, magic formulae, shortcuts, stereotype systems or panaceas. A body doesn't follow systems, formulae or books. There is no disease that follows a fixed pattern.

Each disease is as different, personal and specific as the fingerprint of the one who is ill. Symptoms and formulae have to be adapted to and fixed to the individual, much as tailoring a dress or a suit to fit. To cure disease, the therapy must cure you, according to your personal needs, not those of someone else, not by taking a remedy that worked for somebody else.

Healing needs change, sometimes within days or weeks. Religiously following an original prescription cannot provide for the necessary changes. Prescriptions are not to be considered as carved in stone.

Healing Processes

A well formulated health-restoring program will satisfy and saturate all body and cell needs. As these needs are filled, the amount and doses originally prescribed must diminish. They will become excessive and eventually, will cause a person to feel worse, not better, just like overeating will cause indigestion.

Health-restoring programs strengthen every body organ. These organs will then attack and neutralize the abnormalities and poisons that caused your disease. They will dump them back into your tissues and blood stream. As these toxic irritants contact nerves in that part of your body, they create pain, distress, and new and different symptoms.

The more carefully you follow the original prescriptions and healing routine, the stronger your body fights and the stronger are the reactions. Unaware of this, you may tend to interpret unpleasant changes, discomforts and symptoms to mean your treatment is wrong for you. You may be tempted to quit. Don't. The new symptoms and changes you are experiencing are messages telling you to give your body a rest – a time to catch up with its needs to detoxify and eliminate whatever its abnormalities or poisons.

Healing reactions are not reasons to panic, quit or become discouraged. They are times to call your doctor. Let him/her explain that such reactions are quite normal. They may require immediate modifying and balancing of your original recommendations and therapies. Periodic communication is in order to keep your healing program constantly in balance with your healing needs. Excess treatments unbalance the body.

There are a hundred possible obstacles to healing: every physical, mental, emotional, spiritual abnormality; every stressful condition of your personal life, family life, social, work life and/or environment.

General Therapy Guidelines

Chronic, long lasting, degenerative diseases are complex. Treatments must consider and manage all complexities.

The amounts of any therapy to be taken must always be the smallest amounts that produce the maximum benefits. Never take more than such amounts – or less. To determine the amounts may require a period of trial and error – up and down juggling – as you attempt to tune into your body's needs.

Nature's healers work slowly. Bodies don't cure. They "grow" back to health and this only happens at the normal speed of any growing.

Bodies attack and react in their own individual ways. Even tests and examinations cannot reveal all this. Your doctor cannot know all the ways except from what you communicate to him.

Accurately formulated therapies generally provide definite benefits within a few treatments or within a few weeks or months. If they don't, something is not right. Something has been missed, misunderstood or misapplied. Get back to your doctor.

Even a most judiciously planned therapy may not resolve all the complexities of a complex illness.

Often it is necessary to proceed stage-by-stage, handling only the most serious healing needs at one time. To treat more than this can overload a body's healing abilities and create complications or other problems.

A need for the assistance of other therapists may arise. No doctor has a total understanding of every aspect of the body, mind and emotions, after all they are infinite in scope and nature. Therapies must work together as a team.

To treat independently one or another leaves a danger of omitting some requirement, of overloading, of duplicating or of giving treatments that conflict with one another.

Do not, on your own, take any treatments, vitamins, minerals, drugs or follow diets or therapies. They could conflict with your doctor's program. Let your doctor know every treatment that you are using and everything you are doing.

The Messages of Body Changes

Bodies heal in unusual, sometimes mysterious ways.
Healing is an ongoing, ever-changing, experience. Bodies express their changing needs by symptoms. The nature of all body changes, both the improvements, as well as those that are adverse, provide your doctor with insights on understanding what he/she needs to adjust the treatments and keep them in harmony and balance with your healing processes.

There is wisdom in our body that guides it to not attempt to correct every problem all at once. As each health problem is resolved, the body will focus on and do whatever is required to resolve other needs that were not initially manifested.

Your Prescriptions

It can happen that your therapies do not provide the relief, the progress and wellbeing that you expected, and need. There are several possible reasons for this:

- Your doctor did not clearly understand everything that is going on in your body, and therefore, did not give your problems the precise consideration they needed. This may be because...
    o You did not tell him/her everything that is related to your problem. You may have forgotten some fact of the past that had a bearing on your health condition. Details get buried in one's mind when overanxious, concerned or suffering. As you recall them, express everything – even the details that you may consider unimportant.
    o He or she may have misinterpreted the meanings you gave to your words, or you misinterpreted the meanings of the words he/she used.

It may be necessary to again discuss your whole illness.

- All treatments must be faithfully and carefully followed until all the disease causes are eradicated from your body and all the body's needs are completely satisfied. It can take up to two years for all sick cells to decompose and disintegrate, and be replaced by normal, healthy cells.

Important aids and general counsels

Your first and most important prescription is teamwork and communication with your doctor. Regular communication makes the difference between successful therapy and healing failure.

Whenever a recommended therapy does not create relief, body comfort, improvement or healing as expected, communicate promptly with your doctor before continuing on with that treatment.

Whenever you are confused or there are problems, reactions, marked changes, be they discomforts or improvements in your condition, make a note of and discuss them with your doctor.

Communication should include completing a progress and therapy evaluation questionnaire every six to eight weeks (more often, if you feel the need).

Know your Supplements

Supplements act differently in different people. Their actions vary according to individuality, nerves, glands, stresses, conditions and diets, as well as mental and emotional states.

The difference between vitamins and minerals versus drugs is that vitamins and minerals are tolerated over a very wide range of dosages, while even slightly high levels of drugs can be toxic. Vitamins and minerals have biochemical roles in the body, whereas drugs do not become part of the tissue or biochemical processes.

Vitamins and minerals are nutrients. Drugs are foreign matter in the body, and after they are utilized, they're broken down and usually discharged from the body's systems.

Vitamins and minerals are involved in a wide range of processes in the body, such as converting food into energy and building bones and tissues. The result is they are constantly being depleted in the body and must be replenished.

Vitamins and minerals must be taken for a long time before there is a possibility of having adverse reactions or symptoms. A one-time mega dose of vitamins is not likely to cause the body harm. Children may have adverse effects from ingesting large amounts of iron supplements. The bottom line is that the overwhelming majority of herbs, even in very large dosages, have shown no detrimental side effects.

Can using more vitamins and minerals for your supplementation program be helpful?

Higher dosages of the antioxidant Vitamins C, E and beta carotene result in more protection for the body, in particular damage from free radical molecules. While the RDIs (recommended daily intake) serve as a point of reference, it should be noted exceeding those levels may offer better health protection.

Supplements that perfectly provide the body's needs may not always do this, if not used precisely as your body requires them. You need to know how to use, balance and regulate them. You need your doctor's guidance in order to do this and to assure your healing process.

Supplements that accurately correspond to your body and healing needs may create some strange unexpected changes, discomforts or reactions. You may be tempted to believe that such reactions mean that those treatments are not right or not helping as they should. Don't presume. Call your doctor for an explanation. He or she will need this information in order to obtain a better understanding of how your body works and how supplements work on your body.

With a good treatment, you may feel worse. You are not getting worse – it is the worst that is coming out. They come out, via your bloodstream. The blood toxins affect your nerves. Do not be influenced to stop your therapy. This is the time to let your doctor know of therapy changes. Your remedies may need to be modified or rebalanced. This is sometimes referred to as the "Healing Crisis". In naturopathic medicine, it is referred to as a period in the self-healing process in which the system is cleansing itself of toxins.

You will experience some uncomfortable symptoms as you begin to detoxify towards health and healing. Most common symptoms may include:

- Skin rashes, lethargy, fatigue
- Cold/flu
- Return of specific recent symptoms
- Irregular bowel movements
- Headaches
- Bloating
- Irritability or other mood disorders

When you are given a homeopathic remedy, you may experience a healing crisis, a temporary exacerbation of symptoms that you presently have or may have had in the past. The symptoms of a healing crisis may be the same symptoms associated with the disease and I will elaborate more when discussing homeopathy later in this book.

Antioxidants

Antioxidants keep free radicals from causing too much damage while at the same time helping the body do what it must to survive and thrive.

Antioxidants are the scavengers that protect your body from free radical damage. Antioxidants are those amino acids, enzymes, minerals, vitamins and supplements that prevent or control the oxidative process, which is like rusting the body from inside and outside.

Free radicals are the negative byproduct created when the body produces energy or due to the body's reaction to such things as air pollution, sunshine, diseases, illnesses, food carcinogens like nitrates and smoke from charcoal barbecues, emotional or mental stress, and almost all activities of daily life to one degree or another. They are responsible for the damaging process caused by uncontrolled oxidation and damage cells, as well as weaken the immune system.

A free radical is one or more atoms that have at least one electron missing, which keeps it balanced. Electrons are negatively charged components of an atom. The missing partner creates an unstable atom, which seeks out a component to complete it. This causes a chemical reaction to occur with other molecules or atoms that are attracted to the free radical atom and easily bond with it. This process happens very quickly and can cause a lot of damage to the body. Over time, the body can no longer compensate for this and disease or illnesses manifest themselves. Antioxidants are the street sweepers that keep free radicals from causing too much damage.

Not all free radicals are bad. They help keep your immune system tuned up and running better by destroying bacteria and viruses. Free radicals help produce energy. They are critical for the production of hormones and enzymes. A lot of substances the body needs require the intervention of free radicals. The problem happens when there are too many free radicals and the body's harmonious function is thrown completely out of whack on a cellular level. Many things and processes can cause a lack of antioxidants.

As we age, our bodies produce less antioxidants and our need to take them increases. This slows down the aging process. Aging can result in degenerative diseases and illnesses, as well as things like weakened eyesight and wrinkles. Even though food is the main source of antioxidants, individual needs exceed what food provides us. Aging and the numerous stresses our bodies endure, increase our need for antioxidant supplementation, which detoxifies our bodies.

Here is a partial list of known free radicals: hydrogen peroxide, hydroxy radicals, superoxide, hypochlorite radicals, nitric oxide, single atoms of oxygen and some lipid peroxides.

A few of the causes that create free radicals in the body are: sunshine and radiation and exposure to toxic chemicals like cigarette and cigar smoke; exhaust from trucks and cars. Environmental stressors, such as pesticides and fertilizers entering our food and water. Chemicals in water, whether they be industrial or used for water treatment, such as chlorine and fluoride. All these affect the body and creation of free radicals.

Antioxidants include these enzymes: Superoxide dismutase (SOD), glutathione peroxidase, methionine reductase. Vitamins and minerals with antioxidants: Vitamin A, beta-carotene, Vitamin C, Vitamin E and selenium. The hormone melatonin, produced by the pineal gland in the brain, is a powerful antioxidant. Nutraceuticals antioxidants in foods include quercetin (apple), lycopene (best absorbed from cooked tomatoes with a little olive oil) , lutein (a carotenoid), glutathione (produced in the body) and zeaxanthin (a carotenoid in spinach and okra). They are found in flavonoids (I.e., reserveratrol, catechins, proanthocyanidins, and anthocyanidins) and isoflavones, such as those found in soy products like genistein and daidzein.

More antioxidants you want to check out are: Alpha-lipoic acid, bilberry, Coenzyme Q10, cysteine, melatonin, ginkgo biloba, grape seed extract, and green tea, oligomeric proanthocyanidins (OPC's) like pycnogenol, selenium and superoxide dismutase.

Food sources high in antioxidants include: red grapes, red wines and purple grape juices; yellow and red onions. Raw or very lightly cooked broccoli, cabbage, cauliflower, spinach, okra, beet greens, Swiss chard, watercress. Raw crushed garlic. Fresh vegetables, especially dark leafy green ones. Pink grapefruit. Fresh whole fruits. Extra virgin olive oil (means from the first cold pressing). Those using organically grown olives are tops. Herbs used in cooking like thyme and rosemary. Carrots, pumpkins and sweet potatoes – the deeper the orange color, the more antioxidants they have.

Combinations of antioxidants are now easily available. They combine components that work better together than alone. In addition, they are usually less expensive and easier to take than if you put the products together on your own. Some formulations include zinc and/or other beneficial nutrients.

The critical problem is getting enough antioxidants to protect our bodies and neutralize the free radicals. Our bodies produce them naturally, but the excessive strains of polluted environments and stressful, unhealthy lifestyle choices almost guarantee the body will not make enough of them. Supplementing with a wide variety of antioxidants is one of the best things you can do for yourself each day.

You can...

Focus into and try to become aware of your body.

Listen to its messages. Listen to your intuition.

Use **moderation** in meals, drinks, habits and lifestyle.

Relax, rest and take siestas. Sleep as much as you can. Only during the quietude of sleep does your body perform all its healing processes of healing.

Slow down and live. Take time for reflection. Go into

your inner self, your emotions and your vision of your total self, your dreams and your needs.

Put aside required or impossible to- live-up-to "shoulds", "gottas", obligations and activities, which create tension and stress. Curtail commitments.

Banish worries, anxieties, fears, negative thoughts. Quiet your mind and emotions. Seek conditions of quiet and peace. Release tensions.

Release pent-up emotions and tensions. Let go of your concerns and whatever has been a bother to you.

If you feel inner distress or emotional discomforts, talk out your problems and feelings with a close and understanding friend, relative or anyone who will listen.

Make **lifestyle changes** that favor healing.

- Decrease overloads; cut down on excesses
- Organize your daily obligations; simplify your goals
- Make changes slowly
- Don't force anything, not even therapies

Exercise

Exercise is as important to healing as your food and supplements therapy. For any nutrient or remedy to have a curing effect, it must reach the areas or tissues in your body where your problems need help. They can only be carried there by your blood. Blood circulation is activated by muscle contractions and expansions through exercise.

To not exercise is to vegetate with little circulation and little healing. Exercise and physical activity is 50 percent of body nutrition and healing. Circulation is as important as diet. Nutrients and supplements can only reach the areas and organs of your body where they are needed and make healing possible by being transported there by your blood.

Exercise regularly, easily and without forcing. Brisk walks, deep breathing, bicycling, swimming, yoga, jogging, tennis, skiing, rebounder jumping, or be active in your favorite sport.

Try **physiotherapy, hydrotherapy or massage**. Indulge in a steam bath or sauna.

Think, live and feel positive and maintain positive attitudes and a positive self-image.

Keep joy in your life. Laugh a little every day.

2

Mastering Your Body's Health

- Your abilities and rights to and chances of achieving optimal health are as great as your motivation and determination.
- Health achievers learn to see an opportunity for healing in every distressful state of their health, rather than distress in every health problem.
- It is not the health that you are born with that makes or keeps you a **health master**. It is how you live and what you do with your health.
- If you want to achieve and maintain optimal health, you must be willing to learn how to know yourself, how to assume complete responsibility for everything you do and for yourself, and persevere in working at being healthy.
- In your mind-set of values, health achievement must rank higher than financial achievement.
- Even in this world of distorted values, attitudes, pollutants and civilization, optimal wellbeing and living is still possible.
- You have two choices in life: you can dissolve into the mainstream, or you can choose to be a master and be distinct. To be distinct, be different. To be different, you must strive to be what no one else but you can be.
- Remember, if your mind will conceive it and your heart will believe it, eventually, you will achieve it.

- If you follow the crowd, you will likely get no further than the crowd. If you walk alone, you are likely to end up in places where no one has ever been before.
- Physical and natural laws are as sacred and binding as sacred or moral laws. In order to be cured of any disease – no matter what – one needs simply to be brought within the range of operations of the laws of his/her organism, and to be so related to them that they can work unobstructed.

"Restoring health is employing those means, which when properly used, would have kept a patient from getting sick in the first place." From *Our Health Platform* by J. C. Jackson, MD

Special Recommendations

- At the end of six to eight weeks, send to your doctor a progress evaluation questionnaire that you can find at the back of this book.
- Check for infections, root canals and tooth impactions through **Dental care.** If X-rays are needed, request the small individual plates rather than the mouth single pictures.
- Check **your spine** for possible manipulation needs. All manipulations should be gentle – not forced.
- **Seek counseling,** if you have been unable to overcome fears, stresses, anxieties, grief, angers and hatred.
- **Keep your body free from toxins** and toxic stagnation. There must be as many bowel movements per day as the number of meals you eat.
- **Check bowel movements** for shape, consistency, validity, size and color. Any abnormality indicates inadequate digestion and utilization of your foods and also your food-type supplements and remedies.

- Check **Feet arches.** If they are flat, they imbalance the structure of the rest of your skeleton. This is stress that hampers healing.
- If there is pain, try **acupuncture** before you try drugs.

The ear chart below shows auricular points – the "Shen Men" points that help with emotional problems. Ancient Chinese culture called this point Shen Men or "The Gate of Heaven". Shen Men is a deep, miraculous point that strengthens your overall health, decreases stress and boosts energy.

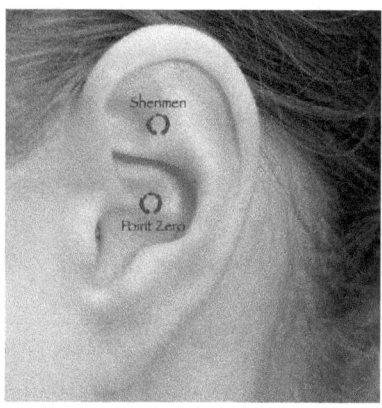

Acupuncture, a 2,500-year-old Chinese practice, aims to unleash the flow of energy, or "Qi" or Chi (pronounced chee) within the body. According to ancient beliefs, disruptions of Qi result in disease and pain. Conversely, a steady flow of Qi brings good health. By probing points of the skin with thin, metal needles, the discipline teaches Qi can begin to flow better. Some Western studies have suggested that acupuncture may stimulate the body's ability to conduct electrical signals and create natural opiods, thereby eliminating some pain.

Understanding Acupuncture

The underlying principles of acupuncture date back

several centuries, when man discovered that hitting the body with sticks, or pressing points on the body with stones, will make the pain go away. Over time, certain points were found to be particularly effective. Based on thousands of years of practical observation and clinical experience, the Chinese developed this into acupuncture, which involves stimulating specific points on the body to treat disease or decrease pain.

Acupuncture may be accomplished by stimulating the points with:

- Pressure - applied with the finger, fruit seeds, stones or other methods

- Hitting - gentle tapping

- Insertion of needles and twirling them with the fingers, applying electricity, light bloodletting or heating with moxibustion (burning herbs attached to the stem of the needle), lamps or lasers

- Cupping - placing small, heated glass jars, which form a vacuum over the points to bring energy to the surface

Traditional Chinese Medicine (TCM) Theory

The traditional Chinese understanding of how acupuncture works relates to *Qi*. *Qi* is the life energy contained in every part of the body. Some *Qi* determines nutrition, helps defenses or helps the blood and circulation, for example. *Qi* must flow around the body harmoniously.

A related concept is yin and yang, the positive and negative aspects or opposing forces in the body, which must be in balance. *Qi* conducts the energy in order to balance the opposing forces throughout the body. A modern corollary for this concept is the sympathetic and parasympathetic nervous system, yielding positive and negative feedback. If *Qi* is in deficiency or excess in any one organ, you get a yin or yang predominant state.

You may have seen drawings showing the meridian lines on the body, depicting where the acupuncture points fall. Each line has a beginning and end, but is linked to another meridian, with the *Qi* flowing in a definite direction. All the meridians are ultimately connected. When the flow is interrupted due to a lack of *Qi* or lack of energy to propel this flow, a pathological condition occurs.

Each meridian line relates to a particular organ, such as the stomach or lungs. Stimulating points along that meridian will help to treat diseases of the organ. The surface acupuncture point on the body is where the internal organ manifests its function. An example of how meridians flow relates to heart attacks, which may cause not just chest pain, but a radiation of pain into the left arm. This arm pain falls precisely along the heart meridian line. Why does needling at a distant point from the problem help? Traditional Chinese medicine theorizes that any one part of the body reflects the entire body. A modern understanding of this might relate to our DNA. Every single cell of our body carries the entire set of DNA codes, thus representing our entire body.

Bear in mind...

No matter what modality is being used by a licensed naturopathic doctor or any other healthcare practitioner, doctors don't heal. They merely provide the guidelines. Only bodies heal. Drugs and chemicals, and chemically processed natural ingredients, don't and can't.

The only supplements that can provide the body's cells with all their biochemical and physiological needs are those extracts from the cells of living plants and beings of nature. Any substance that is chemically extracted and processed, is no longer alive – no longer capable of providing life and healing to the body – is no longer complete and able to totally nourish, replenish and repair cells and tissues.

Do not be misled by the use of the word "natural" on the labels of processed, refined supplements. This word indicates merely that it contains a minimum of $1/10^{th}$ of one percent natural ingredients. This is the law, according to the US Food and Drug Administration.

If every nutrient and condition for healing are provided, and every barrier to healing is eliminated, and if your mind, which is stronger than your body, is normal, relaxed and positive, you can NOT stop your body from healing.

Conclusions and Guidance

- Don't ever force anything. Anything that upsets, stresses or overloads your body must be modified.
- Make changes gradually.
- Use moderation in meals, drinks, habits and lifestyles.
- Banish worries, anxieties, fears and negative thoughts. If you are unable to do so by yourself, get help, counsel and/or support.
- Quiet your mind and emotions. Seek conditions of quiet and peace to help you relieve these tensions.
- Slow down and live. Put aside time every day to relax, reflect, rest and release the effects of your everyday living and any pent up emotions or distresses.
- Do whatever it takes to get enough sleep that leaves you feeling rested, restored, regenerated and more yourself. Only during the quiet of the hours of sleep does your body perform all its processes of healing.
- Make a note of all body changes, improvements, problems, reactions, difficulties or discomforts.

Discuss them on an ongoing basis with your holistic physician.

- Think, live and feel positive.
- Maintain a positive self-image and self-esteem.
- Read positive, morale building, and joy-giving books.
- Keep joy in your life. Laugh a little every day.

Whenever anxieties, concerns and difficulties of your disease become more than you can take, try this magical remedy:

On a good-sized sheet of paper, print four words, then get on your knees, join your hands and fervently say these words: **"To hell with it."**

Do not be offended by these words. Your disease and distresses are like hell in your life. The thing to do is to send them back to where they belong.

When everything is too much for you, it is not time to start dealing with the worries and anxieties of your problems. You can put them back on to your shoulders and try to find solutions for them later when you feel better. Attempting to resolve more than you can handle, when in a serious disease state, can overload and block healing.

3

The Body's Biochemistry

Body biochemistry, acid/alkaline imbalances are not to be treated lightly. One of the first and most basic health-maintaining and/or therapeutic prerequisites is to balance the pH – the acidity/alkalinity of the body.

Acid-Forming and Alkaline-Forming Foods

The comparative qualities of the various foods in this list are indicated by **"X's"**.

1 X = mild, low excesses of acid or alkaline

2 X = moderate levels of acid or alkaline

3 X = strong, high levels

4 X = very strong high acidity/alkaline levels

Acid means acidifying. Some foods are alkaline by nature but, when processed by the body, leave an alkaline influence on the body medium.

Alkaline means alkalizing. Some foods are acid, but when processed, leave an acidic influence on the body.

Many foods of one type, as they pass through our body, are acted upon by the body's chemistry. They produce an acid or alkaline residue opposite to their original chemical composition. Foods that are acid will alkalize and vice versa. To avoid confusion, foods are listed by the impact they leave on the body.

Some foods conflict. Strong acid-creating foods (XXX – XXXX), are obviously antagonistic to strong alkaline-creating foods (XXX-XXXX).

It is best that they not be taken at the same meals. They can mutually interfere with the digestion and assimilation of each other.

Quality, Recommended Foods	Acid	Alkaline
Almonds, unsalted		X
Apples, fresh		XX
Apples, dried		XX
Apricots, fresh		XXX
Apricots, dried		XXXX
Asparagus		XX
Bananas, ripe	XX	
Barley	X	
Beans: navy, baked		XXX
Beans: green, fresh in pods		XXX
Beef	XX	
Beets, fresh		XXXX
Berries, all kinds		XX to XXXX

Cabbage		XXX
Cantaloupe		XXX
Carrots		XXXX
Cauliflower		XXX
Celery		XXXX
Chard		XXX
Cheese: hard, aged	XX	
Cherries		XX
Chicken	XXX	
Corn, dried		X
Cranberries	XX	X
Currants		XXX
Cucumbers, fresh		XXXX
Dandelion, greens		XXX
Dates		XX
Eggs, whole	XXX	
Eggs, whites	XXXX	
Figs, dried		XXXX
Fish	XX to XXX	
Fruits, nearly all		XXX
Halibut steak	XXX	

Quality Foods Cont'd	Acid	Alkaline
Lamb	XXX	
Lamb stew	X	
Lemon juice, natural		XXX
Lettuce		XXXX
Lima beans, dry	X	
Liver, beef	XXX	
Muskmelons, alone		XXX
Mutton	XX	
Oatmeal, cooked	XXX	
Oils, from seeds, grains, nuts	XX to XXX	
Onions		XX
Orange juice, natural		XXX
Parsnips		XXX
Peaches		XXX
Peanuts	XX	
Pears		XX
Pecans	XX	
Peppers		XXX

Plums	XX	
Peas: fresh, green		X
Peas: ripe, dry	XX	
Pineapple		XXX
Potatoes: white (eaten with skins)		XXX
Potatoes: sweet (eaten with skins	X	X
Prunes	XX	XX
Pumpkins, not sweetened		X
Radishes		XXX
Raisins		XX
Rhubarb, high in oxalic acid		XXX
Rye, other seed grain	XX to XXX	
Salmon	XXX	
Spinach		XXXX
Squash, summer		XX
Squash, winter	X	
Tomatoes		XXXX
Tomatoes: canned, no sugar/salt		XXX

Turkey	XX	
Turnips		XX
Walnuts	X	
Watermelons		XXX
Poor Quality Foods to be Avoided		
Bacon, fat	X	
Bacon, lean	XX	
Pork, lean	XX	
Bread: whole wheat, white	XX	
Milk (pasteurized)	XX	
Bread: whole wheat, whole grains	X	
Breakfast foods	X to XXX	
Cheese cottage	X	
Clams	XXX	
Corn Flour	XX	
Cornstarch	X	
Fruits: stewed, sugared	X to XXX	
Grape juice, sweetened	XXX	

Lard		X
Lobsters, Crabs	XXXX	
Milk, whole		XX
Olives: green, pickled	XX	
Oysters	XXXX	
Rice: natural, polished	XX	
Shredded Wheat	XX	
Veal	XXX	
Wheat, whole, cracked	XX	

Note: All animal fats are harmful. Heating them makes them even more toxic. Lard in cooking and frying, and overheated rancid oils makes foods more rancid and more acidic.

Determining pH – Body Acid – Alkalinity

This is done by the use of pH test strips, used on both the saliva and urine; one without the other is inadequate.

Saliva

1. Tear off a short strip from your pH roll.
2. Heavily moisten your tongue with the saliva.
3. Place the pH strip onto your tongue for several seconds – no more, no less.

4. Check the color that appears on your pH strip with that on the pH chart in your pH container.
5. It is best to make a record of the results.

Urine

1. Void a small amount of urine.
2. Make a strip of pH test paper contact the urine – for a second – no more
3. Check color as above.
4. Include this on your record chart.

PH Normal(s)

Saliva =7.0 – 7.4   Urine = 5.0 – 6.0

Too many kinds of foods at one meal add a burden to the digestion.

Alive, green leafy vegetables provide nutrients in a balanced and most easily digested form.

Common factors other than foods that create acid – alkaline imbalances:

- The worst is stress. It exhausts the adrenal glands. A major role of these glands is to control and limit the amounts of alkaline minerals that are flushed out of the body through the kidneys. This can often be recognized by high alkalinity of the urine – a pH higher than 6.5.
- Nervousness, tenseness and anxiousness, worries, anxieties, guilt, angers, foods and insomnia.
- Exhaustion. General exhaustion is also exhaustion of the adrenal glands.
- Excessive intake of high acid foods. Most diets that people consume are up to 90 percent acid foods.
- The failure to include generous portions of alkaline type foods. Alkaline type foods are alkalizing because

they are in the alkaline minerals, mainly potassium and calcium.

- Infections. Any infection whether it is a cold, flu, abscess or infection of any organ, creates states of body acidity. Both saliva and urine will be acid.
- Lack of hydrochloric acid from the stomach. This acid is essential for the digestion of the alkaline foods and the absorption, and utilization of their alkaline minerals because they infiltrate into body fluids and tissues. This is recognized when both saliva and urine turn very acid.

All balances are essential to health and healing. Balance is a major aspect of health. There is no health or healing unless there is chemical balance.

4

Your Body's Healing

Your body never stops healing. It heals constantly.

Do you need a reassurance of that? Then make a slight cut in your skin – anywhere. Protect it from irritation or infection. Put a Band-Aid on it, if you wish. Notice that it automatically heals. In fact, you can't stop it from healing. Of course, if you keep scratching, irritating or infecting it, you may damage the area faster than your healing can repair it.

More subtly, there are quiet songs of increasing wellness that well up inside us. Listen to your body. Have confidence in its healing abilities. When you heal, you feel better.

You feel a little happier. You feel a release from anxieties. There is less tension. You relax better. Your head feels lighter. Your mind works better. You sleep better. You function better. Your body becomes more limber. Your energies are better. Your nerves are less irritated. Aches and pains decline and fade. Skin problems or eruptions will disappear. You start to feel more like your old, natural self. You don't need a doctor or laboratory tests to tell you that you are improving.

Healing is like baking a chocolate cake. You obtain all the specified ingredients (your supplements and remedies). You are given a recipe (your healing counsels and understandings). You mix all the ingredients together exactly as prescribed. You leave it to bake for as long as the recipe calls for. In the same way, you allow your body the weeks, months or years needed for all the remedies to bring about their complete and optimal benefits. Your careful following of the recipe will obtain a chocolate cake – not some other kind of cake. In healing, it is possible only that your body processes reap the benefits of your caring and return to health.

However, your body goes beyond this. Your healing takes place even at times and during periods when you feel worse.

In order to heal, our bodies must get rid of all of the causes of illnesses: the toxins, wastes, poisons, infections, abnormal substances or chemicals, drugs, damaged and dying cells. As soon as it has enough energy and healing power to do this, it attacks them promptly. In the process those foreign substances are thrown into the bloodstream.

Here comes what feels like a problem: a body that pours toxins into the bloodstream undergoes similar reactions to a person who puts poisons in their mouths. The blood goes directly to your brain. Your brain feels it. You may get a headache or feel tired or low or heavy, or miserable. It becomes intoxicated and actually somewhat poisoned by all this refuse. That is until it can be cleared from the blood. When like this, you may feel worse, but you are not worse. It is a sure sign that the "worseness" – the culprits that caused your illness – are being transported to the organs of elimination.

This reaction or hangover, or "drying up" period is generally known as a "healing crisis". When properly caring for most healing crises, they won't last long.

While following a regime that corresponds to your body's healing needs, your body cannot get worse. Worse feelings are the worst coming out, not making worse.

It is not possible to have healing and health

improvement at the same time as your condition is deteriorating or the treatment is backfiring, and not working.

It is not possible to have health and disease at the same time. When you get rid of the abnormalities, which make up the disease, you get better.

It is not uncommon, at some point after the feeling that your condition has completely cleared up, to undergo experiences of an old illness, fever, infection, or health problem that troubled you earlier in life. This only means that all the healing measures that you should have known about and followed at that time were not used. All the causes were not totally neutralized or eradicated. Some of the chemicals or drugs that you may have used are still stored in your body's tissues.

Drugs tend to debilitate and block the organs they affect from getting rid of them completely. Your healing was not complete. Residues of some of that old toxicity or illness are still stagnating in your system. Re-experiencing an old illness does not mean you are getting it again. It means that you are getting at it and getting rid of it.

Healing always takes time. It proceeds at the same speed as growing. Your body heals as fast as it took to grow from being a teenager into becoming an adult. There is no way to make it heal faster than nature can handle.

Getting rid of causes, and replenishing a deficiency or something your body is starved for, can happen relatively quickly. One goes through a feeling of marked improvement and wellbeing at the start of many healing programs. This can be misleading. It leaves the false sense of security that all is now well. If so, then one can phase out all the diet and therapy requirements and go back to living, much as one was accustomed to living before the illness first started. In a sense, this is not really healing. Complete healing is the dying off and ejecting of old sick cells and replacing them with new, young, alive and strong healthy cells.

Happiness

Laughter

Joy of living

Peace of mind

Serenity

Acceptance

It has been said that laughter is the greatest medicine. Don't knock it. Try it. Never underestimate it. It has cured many an incurable disease. These pages are no laughing matter, even though the matter is laughter.

Laughter is a remedy for many ills. It can cure more quickly than the doctor's tiny pill.

If you want to keep your head, your heart and health, it would sure help to laugh your head off.

Life without laughter would be dismal indeed. To brighten your pathway to health, I have assembled here some light bits from the drama of everyday living.

A little ridiculousness is thrown in with the humor in order to counterbalance it. Some of our values of living (those that are doing us in), need to be ridiculed. They aren't funny at all, but we sure should learn to laugh at them.

The way some people behave, you would think being pleasant was hazardous to their health.

"Pure enjoyment through life has more to do with one's healing and happiness, and efficiency than almost any other single element." - George Matthew Adams.

Nature's 18 Greatest Healers

- Faith – believe in the self and body
- Hope
- A life and the purpose to live for
- Loving and being loved
- Appreciation (love lived)
- Joy, humor and laughter
- Power and wisdom of mind
- Positive attitudes
- Positive lifestyles
- Moderation – self-control
- Sleep, rest and relaxation
- Life forces of foods
- Diet and nutrition cell-building materials
- Air, oxygen and deep breathing
- Water
- Sun
- Herbs

No medicine beats laughter as a healer

Laughter is a powerful therapy. Regular doses will keep you healthy. It can even extend your life. At least it will make your life seem longer and greater. It reduces stress and tension, and provides other health benefits.

Your 12 Healing Forces

- Motivation. Willpower. Determination
- Your body's innate wisdom
- First is understanding:
    - Health
    - You
    - The nature of your illness
    - Managing its causes and how healing works

- Endocrine glands
  - Hypothalamus and pituitary
  - Thyroid
  - Adrenal – adrenaline, cortisone
  - Liver - your laboratory of living

- Forces of life
  - Digestive enzymes, which make all forces available
  - Metabolic, catabolic enzymes
  - Enzyme activators; vitamins
  - Vitamins without enzymes. Temporary action

- Blood circulation activators
  - Exercise
  - Magnetism
  - Cell electricity – H CI
  - Laying on of hands

- Cooperation with your holistic physician

Strategies for expanding health and joy

- Give yourself permission to experience feeling good and alive - all the joys and potentials of being you.
- Recognize and accept that you are bigger than your mind and body. Your being embraces a wonderful and broad horizon of heart, feelings and intuition.
- Rather than sitting back and reacting to the world as most people do, create your own joys and potential fulfilling experiences.
- You are the master of your own being, your life and your destiny. Realize and accept that YOU control your life, thoughts and feelings. Do not let them control you.

- Take time, every day, for moments of quiet and solitude. Go into the core and centre of your being.
- Choose and do those things you have always wanted to do – things you have found joyful and fulfilling. Discover your abilities to do them.
- Saturate your life and days with positivity.
- Do the things that are really joy(s) for the real you.
- Don't deprive any ability by not using it.
- Listen to happy, lyrical music.
- Visit your good friends.
- Go dancing.
- Read a good book.
- Meditate. Smell a rose.
- Go into the wilderness; lie on the beach.
- Be positive, live positive, think and choose positive.

I AM THANKFUL I AM ALIVE

A man bought a farm long since grown over with weeds. At the end of a year, a clergyman called and complimented the farmer on how well he and the good Lord had succeeded in beautifying the place; to which the farmer replied:

"Thank you, Reverend and I'm glad you included me, because it sure was a mess around here when the Lord was running it by himself!"

Helplessly, we arrive in this world, add what we can to the general confusion and then depart with equal helplessness. The impression left behind by most of us often just about equals the hole left in a bucket of water after a clenched fist is withdrawn. This is because we cast aside many precious gems of understanding and wisdom – of appreciation of the greatness, wonders, beauties and miracles of all of creation. An objective glance in the mirror reveals one of the beauties of God's creatures and masterpieces.

There isn't a soul who doesn't know in his heart that the greatest satisfaction comes from love for, and service to others. Yet we continue to envy, despise and deceive. We pity, when we should love. We resent and begrudge when we should respect and admire. We are fascinated by gossip, venerate mediocrity and scorn truth, and light. Integrity is for "squares" and is "for the birds".

To each of us, there eventually comes a moment of truth when it becomes remarkably clear that life is a privilege. Life is an opportunity to share in all the marvels of creation.

The object of living is to appreciate. Appreciation is love that is lived: "I am glad that I am me and I'm glad for what has been given to me to be, to live and to offer to life." To the extent that we make use of the faculties with which we are endowed, do we live this glorious experience called life.

PART II

SAD STATES OF MIND

"Every man has his secret sorrows which the world knows not; and often times we call a man cold when he is only sad." — Henry Wadsworth Longfellow

5

Depression

"Depression is the world's most widespread disease. One third of all North Americans wake up depressed every day. Only 10 to 15 percent of people consider themselves happy." - World Health Organization

Depression is often only sadness and melancholy rather than serious inner disturbance or illness. It is a state of mind that focuses on the past – the good old days, the good times. It is believing that all that is past. It is difficult to let go of that past and the youth once lived. There is nothing in the present or future to look forward to.

The Nature of Depression

Basically, depression is neither good nor bad. It is simply a state of being. Often it is a mechanism of body and soul creating such a state in order to force us to put aside our carved-in-stone attachments, attitudes, habits and desires that stem from the past, and induce us to adopt needed valuable changes in growth, thinking, feeling and/or living, and to broaden our vision and mature to greater personal wisdom and fulfillment of neglected potentials and abilities of our natures.

The Negativity of Depression

Depression is a lowered state of body, mind or emotions. The lowering comes from inadequate input or deprivation of the body's needs or from toxicities, which slow down or hamper the organs, nerves and general functioning.

The gloom of depression is actually anger, a frustration over the losses of past pleasures, lifestyles and values to live by – an anger directed inward, because of an unreasonable compulsion not to show it outwardly. An Olympic athlete who loses the use of a leg or a foot will be overcome by the disability and be depressed.

Depression is a lowering of, or deprivation of any natural state or condition of body, mind and/or spirit.

- Vitality
- Morale
- Hope
- Self-image
- Physical health
- Mental health
- Emotional health
- Any dysfunction of an organ

"Depression and anxiety can be the first symptoms of an endocrine gland disorder." - *Newsweek*, Jan. 12, 1987

Anybody who has lost a dear one is deprived of the essentials for living the joys of one's nature.

Anyone who suffers a serious injustice is also a victim of what is required to find joy in life.

Anytime there is anything wrong, toxic, at fault, or deficient in a body, the nervous system transmits a message to this effect to the brain. The nerves do not have words. The message that continues to bombard the brain, until the condition is corrected or alleviated: "Wrong,

wrong, wrong." Eventually the conscious mind takes over and says "I am wrong". I do not know the full nature of the wrong. I am unable to bring everything back to perfection. This demoralizes and discourages. The result is depression.

One of the major patterns of depression is the thought that what was our joy and pleasure of the past will be gone forever. Not knowing what the future will bring leaves souls in remote haunts of emptiness and discouragement. They may feel disillusioned. The values, ideas, convictions and habits by which they lived for years, no longer seem to be, or will be valid.

Depression is the...

- Low, non-living of one's true full self, every deviation from the path to one's fulfillment, when blocked by one's false private self. Not to accept and love, and do God's will is to refuse the fullness of his or her existence.
- Wanting or trying to exist – but not live – outside of reality and outside of life – an illusion.
- Fruits of our disordered desires, which look for a greater reality in the object than what is actually there.
- Seeking greater fulfillments than any created thing is capable of having or others are capable of giving.
- Self-centeredness. Worshiping ourselves.
- Indulging in inordinate self-gratifications.
- Self-hatred
- Masochism
- Closing doors to joys
- Self-pity
- Negative attitudes
- Worrying – mainly about self
- Living the past
- Living in a state of too much inactivity

- Believing false values
- Loss of faith – leaving God out of one's life
- Not realizing or recalling that everything in life goes by cycles, or about the meaning of "Resurrection".

Depressions follow panic, just as surely as a hangover follows excessive drinking. When a human body suffers profound endocrine gland disruptions as a result of a crushing fear or other profound emotional disturbances, depression is an almost automatic aftermath.

"The great tragedy of life is what dies inside a man while he still lives." - Albert Schweitzer

Depression is not a sign of weakness, but a sign of need.

Depression is the effects on our bodies, minds, emotions and soul, of an imbalance between the positive and joyful experiences and the failure to include them in our hearts and lives.

Versus

Happiness, Joys	Shoulds, Gottas
Positives	**Negatives**
Self-fulfilling accomplishments	Accomplishment deprivations
Fulfilling experiences	Traumatic experiences
Enjoyable times	Empty – lonely times
Health-restoring foods	Devitalizing foods
Restful, relaxing times	Overloads, excess work

Sleep	Insufficient sleep
Holidays, days of rest	Constant hyper-activity
Interesting times	Periods of boredom
Love in one's life	Deprivation of love
Gratifying milieu	Depleting milieu
Nourishing environment	Depriving environment

Depression is physical deprivations

1. **Hypoglycemia.** Breakfasts of only sugars and sugar-type foods. Foodless foods supply energy to the body for only about 20 minutes.
   After that time, the body lives on reserve energies. After years of doing this, the reserve energies needed to keep emotions, nerves, organ functions at a normal level, decline. You and your whole body get depressed.

2. **Oils**. Liver, adrenal glands, thyroid, nerves and multiple other functions are made possible only by a generous intake of certain quality oils. These oils are destroyed by the intake of rancid or chemically treated oils and fats – fats of meats, tuna, margarine, sausages, fried foods, commercial salad dressings and oils; oils stored on shelves rather than in freezers.

3. **Poor or insufficient blood circulation.** Lack of exercise and activity. Poor posture. Too much TV. Food can also slow down the blood. More than any other such food is wheat. Many people don't tolerate

it. The gluten thickens the blood the same as making glue when mixing flour with water.

4. **Foodless foods**. Wheat foods, milk, the standard boxed cereals, canned foods (tuna), fast and junk foods.

5. **Lack of proteins.** Proteins are essential to feeling good, being alert and alive. Several of the amino acids sustain morale and vitality. A lack of them can bring depression.

6. **Tired or under-functioning adrenal glands.** These maintain dynamism, energy, vitality, the ability to cope with difficult and seemingly impossible stresses and situations.

7. **Lack of sleep.** The lack of sleep weakens our abilities to cope with our distresses and overloads. The long sleepless hours allow the mind to become overloaded with life's difficulties, stresses, worries and anxieties.

8. **Imbalances of proper ratios** of calcium, magnesium, potassium and trace minerals in the fluids that surround the brain causes an irritation of brain cells with resulting nervousness, impairment and or depression.

Toxicities and Depleting Factors

Toxicities, are like overdoses of alcohol, the after effect is always a hangover which is a depression.

1. **Mercury in the teeth.** Constant drainage of dissolved mercury into the system. Few substances are more toxic than mercury.

2. **Root Canals.** Bacterial infections invade and wall themselves off in the roots of almost all canalled teeth. It is impossible to disinfect them. They become abscesses. The poisons from those abscesses travel into and along the nerves that go to the brain and spinal cord.

3. **Cavitations.** This is a term used to indicate that the jaw bones have been invaded by infections following tooth extractions, which were not done properly or properly sterilized. This is another form of dental abscess. It acts the same as root canals.

4. **Cigarettes.** They are radioactive and full of pesticides and chemicals.

5. **Retained bowel movements.** For every meal there must be elimination, or there is retention. The retained fecal matter is toxic.

6. **Overloaded liver.** All the toxins, including inadequate intake of foods and oils. It cannot function without oils. People with depressed livers are invariably depressed.

7. **Faulty digestion.** Foods that don't digest, rot and putrefy in the bowels. This is very toxic.

8. **Allergies.** Allergens act on the body and on the nerves the same as drugs or poisons. Allergens are powerful irritants. They trigger the nerves to contract blood vessels. This is an attempt to block the flow of the toxic irritants throughout body, brain and nerves. The narrowing or closing of blood vessels markedly lowers the transport of nutrients to all body organs, nerves and brain. This lowers the

flushing out of normal cell and tissue body wastes, toxins and acids. Acids accumulate. Acids are powerful brain and nerve irritants.

9. **Too many tranquilizers and/or sedatives.** Over a period of time, they poison the nerves they sedate. They poison the liver, whose role is to maintain body and mind activity, health and positive attitudes, and to rid our bodies of all forms of toxins chemicals and pollutants.

Constant, frequent stimuli leave the body tired and run down

The aftereffects of all stimulants and every strong, energizing and activating of the body's energies will eventually deplete them. A tired body is like an automobile that has run out of gas. The effect is depression.

- Coffee is a stimulant. It is not possible to continue to stimulate nerves, organs and the body when their reserves are so depleted that they cannot respond. The result is depression.
- The standard vitamins and minerals are stimulants, rather than healers. Their constant use eventually burns up reserve energies.
- Inactivity, sedentary work and living can predispose a body to feel sluggish and eventually depressed.
- Often feeling rotten has to do with the environment you constantly live in.

It should be obvious that no one can live with an accumulation of the above experiences over a period of years and expect the body, mind, nerves and emotions to function on a level of happiness and wellbeing. A body will

Excess Stress Causes Depression

Numerous researches have shown that prolonged stress and specific traumatic experiences change the biochemistry of your brain and your hormones.

In the 1960's, researchers Thomas Holmes and Richard Rahe examined the medical records of thousands of medical patients as a way to determine whether stressful events might cause illnesses. Patients were asked to tally a list of 43 life events, based on a relative score. Their results were published as the Social Readjustment Rating Scale (SRRS). The chart below is more commonly known as the Holmes and Rahe Stress Scale. Additional studies have supported the links between stress and illness.

Life event	Life change units
Death of a spouse	100
Divorce	73
Marital separation	65
Imprisonment	63
Death of a close family member	63
Personal injury or illness	53
Marriage	50

Dismissal from work	47
Marital reconciliation	45
Retirement	45
Change in health of family member	44
Pregnancy	40
Sexual difficulties	39
Gain a new family member	39
Business readjustment	39
Change in financial state	38
Death of a close friend	37
Change to different line of work	36
Change in frequency of arguments	35
Major mortgage	32

Foreclosure of mortgage or loan	30
Change in responsibilities at work	29
Child leaving home	29
Trouble with in-laws	29
Outstanding personal achievement	28
Spouse starts or stops work	26
Beginning or end school	26
Change in living conditions	25
Revision of personal habits	24
Trouble with boss	23
Change in working hours or conditions	20
Change in residence	20
Change in schools	20

Change in recreation	19
Change in church activities	19
Change in social activities	18
Minor mortgage or loan	17
Change in sleeping habits	16
Change in number of family reunions	15
Change in eating habits	15
Vacation	13
Major Holiday	12
Minor violation of law	11

Stress, adrenal exhaustion causes depression

Stress is a challenge that makes us live. Stress can teach us great lessons.

Contrary to all talk and negative ideas about stress, normal stress is not an evil. It is not a threat to our lives or to our health. It does not hurt us. It is harmless. That which is a threat to our lives and does hurt us, is the way we react to stresses. Of course, excruciating stresses can be painful and traumatic. But even they don't have to hurt us, if we learn to react to them in a sensible way.

It even helps us and forces us to live. Without challenges, we would remain weaklings and jellyfish. Without stresses, few of our strengths of character, of our mental and emotional abilities, of our willpower and even of our bodies would never develop, grow, or reach a maturity. We would continue through life like children. It is doubtful, if we would ever really learn to face up to life and the facts of life. As Hans Selye mentioned: "It is not stress that will harm you, but rather, your reaction to stress."

Stress is constant and we are always exposed to it every day. In our fast, bustling society today, we have an incredible amount of stress and our body reacts by mounting a stress response through the stimulation of the sympathetic nervous system. Hans Selye did a lot of research on stress and referred to the "fight or flight" response as the body arms itself to face what it perceives as potential danger. When this happens, epinephrine is secreted from the adrenal medulla, and the hypothalamus-pituitary axis is stimulated to release ACTH, which in turn, causes the adrenal cortex to increase production of the anti-stress hormone cortisol.

The adrenal glands that secrete hormones are walnut-sized glands, located above the kidney and often become 'exhausted' as a result of the constant demands placed upon them. The outer layer of the glands, called the adrenal cortex, produces hormones including cortisol, DHEA, estrogen and testosterone. The function of the adrenal glands is performed by a wide variety of hormones released by the inner adrenal medulla and the outer adrenal cortex, which is mostly directed at the physiological response to stress. The medulla is responsible for producing epinephrine and norepinephrine (adrenaline), which control the body's reaction to stress and affect blood pressure, heart rate and sweating. The adrenal cortex produces hormones such as cortisone and aldosterone which are necessary for fluid and electrolyte (salt) balance in the body as well as regulating the use of dietary protein, fats and carbohydrates and controlling inflammation.

Major health problems can occur when the adrenal glands produce too many or too few hormones.

An individual with adrenal exhaustion will usually suffer from chronic fatigue, may complain of feeling stressed-out or anxious, and will typically have a reduced resistance to allergies and infection. The adrenal glands secrete several important hormones that help maintain the balance of many body functions. Stress, fasting, temperature changes, infections, drugs, and exercise all stimulate the adrenals to release their hormones. When the adrenals release too few or too many hormones, the body responds differently to the everyday stresses of life.

Adrenal fatigue has a broad spectrum of non-specific, yet often debilitating symptoms. The onset of this disease is often slow and insidious. When a person experiences chronic stress, the cortisol level may rise to such a high level that its production reduces as the adrenal glands become exhausted.

Under normal conditions, cortisol helps convert proteins into energy, releasing glycogen and counteracting inflammation. For short durations this is fine, but at sustained high levels, cortisol gradually tears your body down. This leads to the destruction of healthy muscles and a bone, slow down healing and normal cell regeneration, impairs digestion, metabolism and mental function; interferes with healthy endocrine function, and weakens your immune system.

In the early stages of adrenal dysfunction, cortisol levels are too high during the day and continue rising in the evening. This is called "hyperadrenia." In the middle stages, cortisol may rise and fall unevenly as the body struggles to balance itself despite the disruptions of caffeine, carbohydrates and other factors, but levels are not normal and are typically too high at night. In advanced stages, when the adrenals are exhausted from overwork, cortisol will never reach normal levels ("hypoadrenia").

Below lists stressors that can lead to adrenal exhaustion or fatigue.

- Anger
- Chronic fatigue
- Chronic illness
- Chronic infection
- Chronic pain
- Depression
- Excessive exercise
- Fear and guilt
- Gluten intolerance
- Low blood sugar
- Mal-absorption
- Mal-digestion
- Toxic exposure
- Severe or chronic stress
- Surgery
- Late hours
- Sleep deprivation
- Excessive exercise
- Excessive sugar in diet
- Excessive caffeine intake from coffee and tea

When the adrenal glands are not functioning optimally, you can have a condition that is known as adrenal fatigue, or adrenal exhaustion. Adrenal fatigue often develops after periods of intense or lengthy physical or emotional stress, when too much stimulation of the glands leaves them unable to meet the body's needs. The following is a list of symptoms which includes:

1. Excessive fatigue and exhaustion

2. Non-refreshing sleep (you get sufficient hours of sleep, but wake up fatigued)
3. Overwhelmed by or unable to cope with stressors
4. Feeling rundown or overwhelmed
5. Craving salty and sweet foods
6. You feel most energetic in the evening
7. Having sleep disturbances
8. Low stamina, slow to recover from exercise
9. Slow to recover from injury, illness or stress
10. Difficulty concentrating, brain fog
11. Poor digestion
12. Low immune function
13. Food or environmental allergies
14. Premenstrual syndrome or difficulties that develop during menopause
15. Consistent low blood pressure
16. Extreme sensitivity to cold

There are many ways to help with adrenal exhaustion, beginning with a proper medical checkup which includes a physical exam, blood work, saliva testing and/or urine tests.

Maintain the following program:

1. Dietary changes to enrich your nutrition and reduce carbohydrates and stimulants. Always have breakfast and smaller meals with snacks.
2. Stress reduction, including moderate exercise (Tai Chi or Qi Gong) and taking more time for you to relax.
3. Do the things that you enjoy.
4. Get more rest.
5. Avoid coffee or other caffeine containing beverages.
6. Eat early and your last meal should be two hours before bedtime.
7. Have a glass of water (warm) in the morning with ½ squeezed lemon.

8. Avoid grains, such as bread.
9. Avoid starchy foods, such as potato and trans fat (fries).
10. Try laughing yoga and avoid getting over-tired.

As with any specific type of treatment, the treatment(s) for adrenal disease should be based on the underlying cause(s). Treatment generally takes the form of synthetic hormones, which increase the low levels in the body or hormone inhibiting drugs, depending on the disease. Treatment is usually lifelong unless the cause of the disease is removed, such as a tumor which is surgically removed or treated with radiation or chemotherapy.

Due to stressful situations, and an unhealthy lifestyle resulting in adrenal damage and fatigue, it is imperative that this situation be best treated and improved with a holistic and natural approach.

Herbal medicines are well-known for their tonic effect on the adrenal glands and improving the ability to cope with stress. Examples include: Lemon balm, Foti root, astragalus, green tea, licorice root, Ashwagandha, pomegranate, guarana, borage, Siberian ginseng, borage oil. Combinations of herbs with Aswagandha, like Adreanalife, can be used to help deal with stress.

Vitamins and minerals are also needed to help cope with stress, especially the B-complex vitamins and Vitamin C. Antioxidants are also great to provide more energy and slow the affects from free radical destruction. For example, grapeseed extract, pine bark, alpha lipoic acid, omega 3, 6, 9 fatty acids, bioflavonoids, as well as trace minerals, zinc and selenium.

Relaxation methods and reducing stress in one's daily life, as well as eating a healthy, balanced diet and exercising regularly can all be of great benefit to adrenal disease.

Stress on the immune system causes depression

For more than a decade, researchers have known that behavioral and psychological events can influence the immune system. But now new research shows that the immune system sends signals to the brain: "That potently alter neural activity and thereby alter everything that flows from neural activity, mainly behavior, thought and mood," said Maier, professor of psychology at the University of Colorado.

"In a real, true sense, stress makes you physically sick," explained Maier. "In addition, many of the changes over time in mood and cognition from day to day are driven by events in the immune system of which we are unaware. This is a really exciting time for psychoneuroimmunology," "We're finding that products of the immune system alter neural activity and everything else that flows from neural activity. It's not very unusual anymore to think of hormones as regulating neural function, and I believe that in another few years, it will be no less unusual to think of immune products regulating neural function." concluded Maier.

Interesting to note that when I was doing my post graduate studies at Harvard Medical School and later in Chinese medicine, we were taught that emotions are how the body responds to feelings. Traditional Chinese medicine (TCM), view certain emotions which can affect the health of internal organs. Chinese psychology, which is an integral part of traditional Chinese medicine, which has been practiced for more than 5000 years, focuses on the relationship between emotions and organs and their effect on health.

Joy – Sadness   Heart (fire element)

Fear – Fright   Kidney (wood & water element)

Grief – Anxiety	Lungs (metal element)
Anger	Liver (wood element)
Pensiveness	Spleen (earth element)

Joy or Sadness is connected to the heart.
- Joy is an emotion of deep contentment and is connected to the heart, according to TCM. When a person becomes overexcited with joy, it can result in agitation, insomnia and heart palpitations.

Anger affects the liver.
- Anger is an emotion that is associated with resentment, frustration, irritability and rage. This can result in headaches, dizziness and high blood pressure.

Anxiety
- Anxiety affects the lungs and large intestine. This can result in ulcerative colitis and shortness of breath.

Grief
- Grief often occurs when losing a love one for example and affects the lungs. Excessive grief can affect the lungs and cause respiratory diseases.

Fear and Fright
- Fear for example during exams affects the kidneys and causes increased urination. Extreme fear can cause a person to spontaneously lose control of his kidneys and bladder.

Worry and Pensiveness
- Pensiveness is an emotion of excessive thinking and melancholy. It can affect the spleen and cause fatigue, lethargy and inability to concentrate.

Depression Answers and Solutions

All the above need to be corrected, balanced, normalized and restored. Every mental trauma and distress needs positive input, counseling, support of friends, time, change, rest and sleep.

All deprivations and deficiencies need to be replenished. Faulty diets must be replaced with natural, alive, under-cooked, unprocessed and chemically free foods.

Turning towards the future with confidence that everything in life occurs in cycles, rather than focusing on the past and accepting whatever the future may bring, can do a great deal to relieve and forestall depressions.

Circulation deficiencies demand body activity: exercise, deep breathing and freedom from anything that can interfere with the free flow of blood throughout our body, brain and nerves.

All toxic hazards need to be completely eliminated. Mercury amalgams, root canals and cavitations need prompt extraction. They have to be part of the answers.

Other forms of toxins need to be determined and ways found to live free of them.

Depressed people need a lot of emotional and mental support, understanding, counseling and caring, including a patient, empathetic holistic physician.

Stop winding experiences and pleasures, and glories like bandages around yourself, trying to impress others.

Possible Positive Depression Reasons/Answers

In all things, our bodies react to negativities in ways that are positive and beneficial. Every reaction is for a positive purpose and plays a special role.

Depression is no exception. It evokes and awakens the inner core of a person's nature: thoughts, feelings, purpose for living that have been dormant, maybe up to that time over a lifetime. Suppress the depression and you will suppress the undercurrent of the soul's forces striving to come alive and be guideposts to better thinking, feeling and living.

Rolling with the depression puts a reflection on it to analyze it in depth and gives rise to self-understandings, and to the soul's insights, not possible in any other way.

It is important in depression to often recall to mind that life was never intended to be one constant playground or permanent state of happiness, cheerfulness and pleasure.

Depression is like a distiller that works all past and unpleasant experiences, and living into new, higher and more realistic positive levels.

Such reflections can and will (if you let it) bring up buried wisdom – buried aspects of one's nature that have not been looked at, understood or accepted, and lived. All such reflection leaves a person more mature, wiser and more open in mind and emotions.

Guidance and Remedies for Depression

- Seek counsel and guidance.
- Talk to a good friend or close confidant.
- Draw as much strength as you can from others – from loved ones. No one can overcome a depression alone.
- Don't give in to self-pity, self-lowering.
- Don't hold problems and depression inside.
- Learn from others who have known depression.
- Don't allow yourself to get bored.
- Do whatever it takes to restore your optimal health.
- Go on a fast. Detoxify your body.
- Unless your problem is extreme, don't use drugs.
- Never allow yourself to become overtired.
- Never allow yourself to get overburdened.
- Add every enjoyment you can to your living.

- Do something for or render a service to somebody else.
- Listen to beautiful music – your favorite melodies.
- Take time with and play with children.
- Reach for another. Listen to somebody else's troubles and sorrows.
- Undertake a difficult task or challenge.
- Smile a little every day, even if you have to force it.
- Remember that nothing is permanent or lasts forever. Everything in life goes by cycles.
- Never forget that every difficulty, sorrow and sickness is a blessing in disguise.
- Read uplifting books.
- Draw close to your God.
- Let go and let God.
- Realize that there is no incurable condition.
- Soothe your soul with quietude in nature.
- Be good to yourself.

Affirmation: *The seeds of my own identity, reality, fulfillment and perfection are those that come under the disguises of joys and happiness.*

To maintain inner happiness and peace requires that we maintain close attention, at every moment, to reality and to fidelity of our true natures.

The Hidden Pearls of Depression

Depression can be valuable tools for learning – learning our limits, our inappropriate values we have always lived by in the past, the limitations that wrong ideas, assumptions and attitudes have imposed upon us. While our daily outer living is experienced as negative and deprived, inner workings of the soul may be positive and most valuable as instruments for creating a new life. What looked and felt so good of the past, in a new awareness, may come to our realization as quite superficial, empty and inadequate.

HOW TO FEEL BETTER WHEN YOU ARE DOWN IN THE DUMPS? SUGGESTIONS AND RECOMMENDATIONS

You can make yourself feel better.

- Ask yourself what activities used to make me happy? Have you stopped these enjoyments in your life? Are you starved for joys of living?
- Ask yourself what makes you feel rotten, then do something about it. Learn to understand the causes of your problems by rereading the above conditions.
- Select one or more of those past enjoyments and start doing and living them again. To get started, you may have to make determined decisions and force yourself. Give yourself a pat on the back, or maybe even a little loving kick in the pants.
- Avoid all that is not normal, natural, and health-restoring or that fails to invigorate.
- Try some form of physical activity or exercise, especially a sport or entertainment that particularly pleases you: bicycling, running, swimming, rope skipping, walking – anything, but do it.
  All exertions increase circulation to your brain, nerves and endocrine glands. A body humming at top level counteracts depression. A revitalized body relays a message to your brain which says: "I feel terrific; I feel great". And so will you feel the same.
- Enjoy a particularly satisfying, gratifying food, but one that contributes to health and is part of a well balanced diet – something like an ice cream made from frozen bananas and your favorite frozen fruit, such as strawberries, pears or other berries. Add a little maple syrup and natural vanilla.
  There must always be a protein at every breakfast,

even if it is only a handful of almonds. NO milk, foodless foods, cigarettes, stimulants, coffee, margarine, fatty foods or fish, pork, fried foods and synthetic foods.

- Write down how you feel after each enjoyment you favor: how your body feels, your mind, your emotions.
- If you are still or often tired, indulge yourself with a day (or as long as you can)of relaxing and cozying in bed and enjoy it.
- A change of environment is needed and can be great. Get into a new environment or into a new experience. Go to a concert or a museum.
- Go for a long day close to Mother Nature – a walk through wilderness areas, or a long trip on a lake. Relish her beauty, her quiet and peace.
- Take a trip or a holiday at a place you have always wanted to see or where you have great friends, or where enjoyment is always at its peak, like a Club Med adventure.
- Let your mind escape from your negative feelings and preoccupations. Try a good book, particularly a humorous book. Go to a movie or watch an interesting TV show.
- Call up a friend or acquaintance. Get your mind into a different space of your every day depressed living.
- Get mercury fillings taken from your teeth, if possible. Root canals need to be extracted.

The following questionnaire is a means of acquiring awareness of why you are depressed, what are the causes and how to understand the number of influences in your life that have accumulated to a point where your morale has broken down. Enter a checkmark into the spaces to the left.

Unsatisfied Needs – Something Lacking

___ Anything wrong or negative with my body, mind or life?

___ Anything wrong or seriously lacking in my environment or home?

___Anything that is depriving me of peace of mind or happiness?

___Is there emotional starvation?

___Is there absence of affection and friends?

___Am I being rejected by loved ones?

___Is there an absence of appreciation, respect from friends?

___ Is there a lack of human contact and of an opportunity to express myself?

___Have I had failures in business(es) or enterprises?

___Are there unfinished business and tasks?

___Do I have nutritional deficiencies, starvations?

___Is there a loss of or lowering of energies?

___Is there lower levels of energizing factors:

__Hydrochloric Acid?

__ Enzymes?

__ Alive foods; food sources of energy?

Depressive Attitudes

___Am I not feeling for anyone or anything?

___Am I too dependent on others?

___Have I lost my desire to live?

___What are my disappointments?

Emotional and External Causes

___Hopelessness

___I have an inability to continue to live the good things of the past.

___Grief and losses

___What are my fears, anguish worries and anxieties?

___Do I fear the future and death?

___Do I fear diseases – cancer, AIDS, etc.?

___Do I fear having an illness called "incurable"?

___Do I have a loss of memory and/or mental agility?

___Do I fear abandonment, isolation or loneliness?

___Is there an absence of sharing interests, ideas, activities or dreams?

___Has there been a lot of uprooting and change in domicile and lifestyle?

___Have I had to move into a home or apartment below my social status?

___ Have I retired with lack of obligations, old routines and regular activities?

___ Have I lost a purpose of life or living?

___Has there been a decrease of and/or insufficient

income?

___Is there a lack of religious/spiritual ties (indifference, abstentions)?

___ Are there difficulties falling asleep and/or a persistence of insomnia?

___Am I consistently involved in arguments and humiliations?

___Have I experienced a loss of things that have special value to me: belongings, precious souvenirs?

Awareness of the state of our world and/or the state of others

___Am I disillusioned with political depravities and injustices?

___Am I upset and disillusioned with economic disasters and injustices?

___Am I upset and disillusioned with ecological disasters and hazards?

___Have I experienced injustices of any kind?

___Am I adverse to environmental circumstances?

___Am I experiencing excessive personal difficulties?

___Am I experiencing excessive responsibilities or overloads?

___Am I failing to take time to appreciate the good and the beauties of this world and this life?

Toxicities

___Have I failed to neutralize, catabolize, detoxify and

control my body's toxicities?

___Am I ingesting or in contact with toxic substances?

___Am I retaining, failing to eliminate toxins, and therefore, experiencing constipation?

___Do I have addictions? Taking "kick" drugs?

___Do I have side effects from taking stimulants?

___Am I experiencing alcoholism?

___Do I have allergies?

___Do I have faulty digestions with gas and cramps?

___Do I crave and have many sweets, fats, fried foods?

___Do I yoyo diet?

___Do I eat an excessive amount of junk, dead, foodless foods?

___Do I feel poisoned by foods?

___Do I have mercury filled teeth or root canals?

___Am I experiencing toxins, carcinogens from cancer or AIDs, or arthritis, etc?

Physical Depressants

___My body is aging and I feel a loss for my youth.

___My loss of beauty by a disfigurement.

___Do I have an ongoing, serious illness?

___Am I experiencing pain, distress and discomforts?

___Have I lost some of my physical or mental abilities and

functions? Inability to perform usual or ordinary tasks?

___Am I sedentary? Not exercising or doing physical activities?

___Have I lost a limb, organ, hearing or sight?

___Do I have deformities?

Depressing Experiences

___Am I feeling blue or low?

___I just don't care anymore?

___Am I waking up with the morning "blahs"?

___Do I have a loss of appetite?

___Nothing tastes good anymore?

___Have I lost my interests and enjoyments?

___Have I lost interest in pleasing others?

___I don't feel like doing anything.

___I don't want to see my friends.

___I don't feel like indulging in my normal or favorite activities.

___I don't want to listen to my favorite music or watch my favorite movies or TV shows.

___I have little desire to smile, because smiling is difficult.

___I feel like God doesn't love me anymore, or care. He has forgotten me or passed me by.

Low Functioning Organs and Glands

___Liver, the organ that creates energy vitality.

___Adrenal glands that help us cope, accomplish and get things done.

___Low thyroid – slow metabolism.

___Faulty gall bladder – gall stones

___Hypoglycemia

6

Pharmaceuticals VS Natural Therapies

There are over 10,000 scientific studies that have been published, documenting natural medicines as safe and effective alternatives for treating diseases and illnesses. Around the world, billions of people use daily safer, successful and inexpensive natural medicines.

Indeed, if one is diagnosed with a mental disorder or other health related problem, one has a choice to choose pharmaceutical therapies. However, there may be natural choices one can consider first, and working with your healthcare practitioners, help mitigate some of the underlying causes and etiologies that are causing emotional problems. As with any drug, natural supplements should be used wisely. Work with your physician or naturally orientated healthcare practitioner for your beneficial quest for optimal health and healing.

Generally, pharmaceutical drug therapies stress your liver, kidneys, digestive system, and body in general, mainly suppressing symptoms; not evoking a healing response and causing many negative side effects.

Natural remedies work in partnership with the body, helping promote the body's own wisdom to heal itself. Natural remedies may offer relief of symptoms. The key is to give the natural remedy and your body enough time to foster and see the healing response.

A rough rule of thumb is that for every year a condition has been developing, it takes one month for a healing response to be evoked. Most diseases and illnesses developed over long periods of time, going from a short term acute condition, to a long-term potentially chronic or permanent condition.

The following examples are in no way complete representations of all the drug or natural remedies and available supplement choices. These examples are a starting point for you to practice the art of self-care and healthcare intervention with your healthcare practitioner.

Anxiety/Insomnia

There are indeed a lot of pharmacological drugs, such as benzodiazepines (Valium, Xanax) to help, but there are potential side effects. The side effects include: allergic reaction, blurred vision, constipation, dizziness, drowsiness, headache, high blood pressure, impaired coordination, indigestion and lethargy.

Natural Choices: There are many herbals to consider, such as: chamomile, kava kava, St. John's Wort and Valerian to name a few. In addition, vitamins and minerals can benefit, along with nutraceuticals.

Potential side effects: kava kava, St. John's Wort, valerian and passion flower are not recommended during pregnancy, unless under professional healthcare supervision. St. John's Wort should not be taken at the same time as antidepressants, unless under medical supervision and it can also make one sensitive to sunlight (photosensitivity).

Ashwagandha (Withaniasomnifera), also known as Indian ginseng.

Biochemical components: Withanolides

What it does: Anti-inflammatory.

It is often used in the Indian Ayurvedic medicinal system to treat many ailments and its health promoting wide range of beneficial effects on the body's systems gives it a reputation as a tonic, reputed to increase physical and mental abilities. It is referred to as an adaptogen due to its ability to help the body adapt to and deal with highly stressful situations.

Withaniais is used for patients with nervous exhaustion, insomnia, debility due to stress, and as an immune stimulant in patients with low white blood cell counts.

Ashwagandha has been used as an adaptogen, diuretic and sedative, and is available as a dietary supplement. It is used in dosages of 450 mg to 2g, in combination with other preparations. *Withaniasomnifera* has been used by Ayurvedic doctors and indigenous medical systems for over 3000 years. There are several showing the clinical trials support the use of *Withaniasomnifera* for anxiety, inflammation, Parkinson's disease, cognitive and neurological disorders and as a useful adjunct for patients undergoing radiation and chemotherapy.

Chamomile (Maticariachamomilla) also spelled Camomile. Biochemical components: Bisabolols, flavonoids, volatile oil. Principal health related actions: anti-inflammatory, antispasmodic, anti-infective, calmative, mild sedative

Suggested uses: To reduces anxiety and inflammations of the mucous membrane. Beneficial for prevention of migraines. Good cleanser for those who have had sustained drug use. Calms nerves. Calms upset stomach. Soothes ulcers. When externally used as a poultice, it has a cooling effect.

Precautions: Those with a severe hypersensitivity to ragweed pollen, rare cases of allergic reaction have been noted. In large doses, it acts as an emetic that does not depress the system.

Damiana (Tuneraaphrodisiaca) Source: leaves and flowers Biochemical components: flavonoids, glycoside, hydroquinone, volatile oil. Principal health related actions: antidepressant, aphrodisiac, nervine and tonic.
Suggested uses: General tonic and relieves anxiety.

Siberian Ginseng (Eleutherococcussenticosus)

In the Chinese healing system, it is used as a warming herb. It is a relative of ginseng. Its calming properties make it the top Chinese remedy for insomnia. Principal body system(s) and part(s) it benefits: Circulation, heart, lungs and nerves.
Properties: Antispasmodic, cardiac tonic.

Suggested uses: Excellent for insomnia. Used as a treatment for arthritis. Beneficial for chronic lung problems and bronchitis. Aids low blood oxygen levels and used to treat stress.

Dosage: A mild herb that requires large amounts to be effective, depending on how bad is the ailment, up to 30 grams daily. When the leaves are used, much less is needed, since they are much stronger. Use between three to eight grams daily.

Hops (Humuluslupulus)
Principal body system(s) and part(s) it benefits: Nervous system, gastrointestinal system.
Principal health related actions: Anodyne, diuretic, hypnotic, sedative, febrifuge and tonic.

Suggested uses: Calms the body down. Stimulates appetite. Relieves cramps, muscle spasms and gas. Alleviates indigestion. Helps alleviate excess water retention problems. Use to treat insomnia, nervous diarrhea and restlessness.

Dosages: To aid digestion, drink a cup of cold hops tea an hour before meals. Excellent after dinner time tea. Mix one-to-two teaspoons in one cup of warm water. Available in capsules and follow label directions. Make a hops pillow to aid in sleeping. Sprinkle alcohol over hops, then fill a pillowcase or small cloth bag with it. Cautions: Prolonged use or excessive dosages should be avoided.

Kava Kava (Piper methysticum)

Principal body system(s) and part(s) it benefits: Kidneys, liver, nerves.
Principal health related actions: Analgesic, antiseptic, antispasmodic, diuretic, aids sleeping, stimulant and tonic.

Suggested uses: Since 1990, Germany has approved kava kava for anxiety disorders. Non-addictive, natural relaxant. Helpful for dealing with insomnia and getting a deep restful night's sleep.

Cautions: Not recommended for pregnant women, lactating women and Parkinson's disease sufferers.

Ginkgo Biloba
Biochemical components: flavoglycosides, quercetin and proanthocyanidins. Contains terpenes.
Principal health related actions: anti-asthmatic, bronchodilator, platelet activating factor (PAF) inhibitor.

Suggested uses: For improved memory: Alzheimer's disease, memory loss, cerebral vascular insufficiency and inhibits blood clotting. Neutralizes free radicals. Beneficial for asthma, stress, tinnitus and vertigo.

Precautions: Take with food. Possible drug interaction with Aspirin and Warfarin.

Oats (Avenasativa)
Biochemical components: Avenacosides, c-glycosyl flavones, proteins and beta glucan.

Principal health related actions: Anti-depressant, cardiac tonic, nervine.

Suggested uses: Debility, depression, menopause symptoms and stress. Excellent natural relaxant, the extract calms the body. To reduce cholesterol by 10 to 15 percent, eat two-to-four ounces of oat fiber each day. This makes it a good preventative measure for heart disease.

Dosages: For external preparations, the oat straw (stalk) is used and it is an excellent source of B vitamin. It is great in regular, foot and salts baths. Oat fiber is available in foods. Try an extract to alleviate the symptoms of indigestion, take five to 20 drops, up to three times a day.

Cautions: Take your time. Gradually increase the amount of fiber you eat. Give your body the time it needs to adjust to this powerful health promoting change. Taking too much at once and bloating, cramps and gas may result - but this too shall pass.

St. John's Wort (Hypericumperforatum)

Biochemical components: Flavonoids, glycosides (hypericin), essential oil.

Principal health related actions: Anti-inflammatory, anti-depressant, anti-anxiety, astringent and sedative. New research indicates its anti-depressant benefits are due to its serotonin reuptake inhibitor properties (SSRIs), meaning it keeps the serotonin levels more constant, which is what Prozac does.

What outsells Prozac, one of North America's top selling anti-depressants, by more than 20 to 1 in Europe? According to the highly respected investigative TV show 60 Minutes, St. John's Wort is used by psychiatrists and other mental healthcare practitioners throughout Europe, more than any other anti-depressant. It is a perennial with regular flowers, which blooms during the summer months. It contains many active ingredients including pseudohypericin, hypericin, xanthrones and flavonoids. Xanthrones and hypericin contain monoamine oxidase (MAO) inhibitors that slow the breakdown on neurotransmitters: norepinephrine and serotonin in the brain. Too much serotonin makes people obsessive and anxious, while too little is thought to be a major cause of depression.

Clinical trials with hypericin extract showed improvement in alleviating the stressful results of depressive symptoms such as anxiety, apathy, insomnia and depression. Add to that the wound healing and anti-inflammatory properties that current research into flavonoids is showing, and the possible anti-viral properties of hypericin and pseudohypericin and you have a powerful healing plant. One of the greatest benefits of St. John's Wort, is that it appears to have none of the side-effects of pharmaceutical drugs.

Suggested uses: Excellent anti-depressant, reduces stress, anxiety and irritability. The ointment alleviates rheumatism and back pain, promotes a restful night's sleep. Supports immune systems associated with antiviral infections and AIDS. Excellent anti-inflammatory and beneficial on dry skin. The oil is used for burns and skin irritations since it has antiseptic and painkilling properties. Researchers at New York University have found it has retro virus inhibiting properties - AIDS virus, HIV, and in animals.

Dosages: For external applications on the skin, use St. John's Wort oil. For mild to moderate depression, 300 milligram (mg) capsule or tablet containing a standardized extract of 0.3 percent hypericin, three times a day. This gives you 1 mg of this herbs' main active ingredient daily. New research indicates severe depression in patients, not suffering delusional or psychotic symptoms, have effectively been treated with double the dosage.

Cautions: Hypericin can make the skin photosensitive. Avoid excessive exposure to sunlight. Safe for humans. Mild reversible side effects have occurred in some users, ranging from gastrointestinal complaints, allergic reactions and or other symptoms. Compared to prescription antidepressants, the amount and severity of side effects is negligible. Commission E, Germany's herb regulatory body endorses St. John's Wort use for depression. When using this herb for long term relief of depression, as a substitute for another anti-depressant or to treat any serious emotional state, I recommend you get professional medical help and supervision.

Valerian (Valerianaofficinalis)
Biochemical components: Glycoside, essential oils, valerenic acid, sesquiterpenes.
Principal body system(s) and part(s) it benefits: Heart, liver, nervous system.

Principal health related actions: Antispasmodic, anodyne, carminative, hypnotic, nervine, hypotensive, sedative and stimulant.

Suggested uses: Beneficial for insomnia, nervousness, anxiety, panic attacks and times of extreme emotional stressful feelings. Balancing agent for exhaustion and hyperexcitability. Alleviates gas, pains, spasms and other general conditions due to stress, such as muscle cramps due to PMS and menstrual cramps.

Dosage: Tablets or capsules, take 1 up to 3 times a day. Liquid extracts or tinctures, usually 5 to 15 drops in water or juice daily, or as per label directions.

Cautions: Avoid high dosages over long periods of time. Not recommended (contraindicated) during pregnancy.

Discover the versatility of herbs

Use herbs as stress busters. The following formulas are usable, if you buy dried herbs. If bought in a prepackaged state, follow the directions on the bottle, unless your healthcare provider says otherwise.

Hops promote relation. Mix 1/2 teaspoon in 1/2 cup of distilled water. Drink daily. You can sprinkle hops on your pillow.
Passionflower is great for times of acute anxiety. Mix 15 to 60 drops of extract in a liquid. Drink daily. Not recommended during pregnancy.

Valerian is known as Mother Nature's own tranquilizer. Take one to three capsules daily or 10 drops of extract in liquid.

Skullcap is a very old remedy for stress. Make a home brewed tea with it - put 1 teaspoon of dried herb in 1 cup of hot water. Mix 3 to 12 drops of extract in liquid, take daily. Take 1 capsule 3 times daily.

If insomnia a problem...

Stress can be one of the underlying causes of not being able to get to sleep. Try an herbal sleep formula in teas, tinctures, extracts or capsules. They are available in most health food stores. The preferred one combines balm, hops, chamomile, oats, passionflower and valerian.

Valerian itself, is one of the best sleep herbs. It reduces activity in the central nervous system. Try it alone if the herbal formulas don't work.

Hops are a sedative and digestive tonic, which may also help you relax. You can get dried hop flowers, put them in an air permeable bag and place under your pillow.

Siberian ginseng is known as one of the best herbal tonics. It also appears to be a cure for insomnia.

Is fatigue a source of stress? Use herbs to reenergize. Try these...

Cayenne's mildly stimulating properties may help. Try a cup of cayenne tea.

American, Panax or Siberian ginsengs, if taken constantly can help eliminate fatigue.

Schizandra is a Chinese herb believed to increase stamina and energy.

Ma huang (Ephedra) is a long acting stimulant. A cup of ma huang tea is said to perk you up.

Ginkgo Biloba is not so quick a mood elevator. The active ingredients in this herb, increase oxygen uptake and blood flow. Alleviating stress-producing symptoms by improving problems, such as memory loss, depression, brain function, as well as cerebral and peripheral circulation. It may take a few days to weeks before sufficient amounts of the active ingredients, ginkgolides and heterosides, are in enough abundance in your body to cause the wanted results. Suddenly, you may realize symptoms have disappeared or been alleviated. Some conditions it may help include: Alzheimer's disease, impotence, asthma, tinnitus, heart and kidney disorders, and your body's ability to utilize glucose.

Nutraceuticals - 5 HTP

Nutraceuticals are substances from natural sources that can have a positive effect upon one's health. These unusual healing products are not herbs, minerals or vitamins. In the proper dosage and concentration, they may stimulate and support the body's healing process. It is their wide range of effectiveness and safety that offers benefits for a variety of health conditions. Properly used, they can eliminate the need to use prescribed drugs, and most importantly the potential negative side effects prescription drugs can cause.

5-HTP - natural antidepressant, appetite suppressant and sleeping aid. The active ingredient comes from the griffoniasimplicifolia, a small bean or seed harvested in Western   Africa.

Biochemical components: 5-HTP (5-hydroxtryptophan) is an amino acid that easily crosses the blood-brain barrier and is then naturally converted into serotonin. Boosts the length of time the levels of the neurotransmitter serotonin stay active in your brain.

Principal health related actions: As a neurotransmitter, it is a calming neuro-nutrient and mood enhancer. Aids sleep. Stimulates platelet aggregation and regulates smooth muscle function in the gastrointestinal and cardiovascular system. Beneficial for relief of chronic pain. Decreased serotonin levels can cause many disorders: anxiety, depression, insomnia, obsessive compulsive disorders (alcoholism, eating, gambling), seasonal affective disorder (SAD), and migraine headaches.

Suggested uses: To normalize serotonin levels in the body. Clinical studies indicate 5-HTP has comparable or superior ability to anti-depressants in treating obsessive compulsive disorders and endogenous depression. In people suffering from insomnia it promotes sleep. Serotonin is the satiety neurotransmitter, shown in psychological and biochemical studies to control eating behaviors.

Suggested dosage ranges: 5-HTP is more beneficial when taken with 50 mg of Vitamin B6, 100 mg of Vitamin B3, 250 mg of magnesium citrate or glycinate. More effective when taken on an empty stomach. Some individuals may need to use 50 mg of pyridoxine-5-phosphate, the active form of Vitamin B6. To treat depression or control appetite, take 50 to 100 mg of 5-HTP a half hour before each meal, three times a day. For insomnia, take 50 to 200 mg 30 minutes before bed time on an empty stomach.

Cautions: Do not use antidepressants and 5-HTP at the same time. 5-HTP produces a few side-effects. Individuals consuming high levels have reported constipation, headaches and nausea. It is not recommended for children, lactating or pregnant women. Persons having a medical condition or taking medications that affect the central nervous system, especially MAOI anti-depressants, alcohol and weight loss drugs, should see their doctor before using 5-HTP. Too much 5-HTP can cause "Serotonin Syndrome", which is an excess of serotonin in the system. The symptoms are agitation, confusion, lethargy, muscle jerks, sweating and tremor. If they appear, immediately stop taking 5-HTP and consult with your naturopath or holistic doctor.

L-theanine was discovered as a constituent of green tea in 1949, and was approved in Japan in 1964 for unlimited use in all foods, including chocolates, soft drinks, and herb teas.

General uses: L-theanine may help relieve stress by inducing a relaxing effect without drowsiness, unlike many pharmaceutical drugs which have many unwanted side effects.

Dosage: Studies reporting an anti-anxiety effect used single doses of theanine 200 to 250 mg.

Side effects: There are few adverse reactions that have been reported in human studies, using tea extracts: headache, dizziness, and GI symptoms.

Toxicities: Theanine is sold in the United States as a dietary supplement and has been granted GRAS (generally recognized as safe) status by the Food and Drug Administration.

Rhodiola Rosea may have beneficial effects in managing mild to moderate depression and mental fatigue. Results from trials evaluating adaptogenic properties and physical endurance are equivocal.

Dosages: used are commonly 200 to 600 mg/day. For depression, doses of 340 to 680 mg/day of R. rosea extract (as SHR-5) have been evaluated for up to 12 weeks.

Rhodiola has adaptogenic effects and has been suggested for improving mental and physical performance through stimulatory effects on various physiological systems.

In lower doses, R. rosea stimulated norepinephrine, dopamine, serotonin, and nicotinic cholinergic systems in the CNS. A double-blind, randomized clinical trial of R. rosea conducted over 6 weeks in 89 patients with mild to moderate depression confirmed potential anti-depressive effects compared with placebo, as measured on the Hamilton Depression Rating Scale, as well as the Beck Depression Inventory. (Darbinyan V, Aslanyan G, Amroyan E, Gabrielyan E, Malmstrom C, Panossian A. Clinical trial of Rhodiolarosea L. extract SHR-5 in the treatment of mild to moderate depression. Nord J Psychiatry. 2007; 61(5):343-348.)

Melatonin is a hormone produced in your brain by the pineal gland. During sleep, the amount of melatonin increases and during the day it falls. It appears to be a master hormone, controlling the circadian rhythm, our body's 24 hour sleep/wake cycle. Around our mid-forties, the reduction in the pineal glands production of melatonin becomes noticeable, as our sleep patterns change. It is a powerful antioxidant that protects cells from the damage free radicals cause.

Potential health benefits: Treatment for jet lag. May be an anti-aging supplement that reverses signs of aging, in turn increasing the quality and length of life. Melatonin offers relief to some sufferers of cluster headaches. It prevents the formation of the amyloid plaque, which kills brain cells and can lead to Alzheimer's disease. Increases immune system functioning. In tests with melanoma skin cancer patients, after the surgical removal of metastasized tumors, the placebo group had a significantly lower survival rate than those given 20 milligrams of melatonin each night. Major benefits of melatonin are that you wake up without feeling groggy and that it is not addictive, like most of the over the counter drugs for sleeping.

Dosage(s): To get a better good night's sleep, or for insomnia, try 1 mg. of melatonin a half hour before going to bed. If that is not enough, then increase the dosage by 1 mg each day, up to a maximum of 4 mgs. The sublingual (under the tongue) type is faster acting, since the melatonin gets into the blood stream, through the mouths mucous membrane, much more quickly.

To prevent the side effects of jet lag, traveling through many time zones, once you arrive at your destination, take 1 to 3 milligrams of the sublingual form of melatonin, about 30 minutes before you want to go to sleep.

For melatonin's cancer fighting properties, under your doctors or natural healthcare provider's supervision, you may want to try 10 to 20 mg. a day of melatonin taken sublingually

Over 40 years of age, take .5 to 1 milligrams before going to sleep, for its powerful anti-oxidant and anti-aging properties.

Caution: Do not drive or operate heavy machinery, if you have just taken melatonin. Do not take melatonin if you are suffering from an auto-immune disease. If you are taking medications, speak with your doctor and tell your pharmacist before taking it, since it can interact with tranquilizers, anti-depressants and other drugs.

Methionine (S-adenosyl methionine-SAM) is an anti-inflammatory, anti-depressant and liver detoxifier. It may be an anti-aging substance, as well as helpful for rheumatoid arthritis, mild depression, liver congestion and many other health problems. It is not toxic.

Methylsulfonylmethane (MSM) is organic sulfur, an essential non-metallic mineral, found in every cell, critical for almost all bodily functions. It is nonallergenic, whereas synthetic, man-made sulfa drugs may cause allergic reactions. The body uses it for the production of antibodies, enzymes, amino acids; a powerful anti-oxidant glutathione, hair, skin, nails, and connective tissue such as collagen and cartilage. MSM is critical to protein synthesis and stability.

Potential health benefits: Very effective in treating strong symptoms of allergic reactions and asthma; promotes wound healing, since it helps connective tissue formation, and thereby, helps skin renew itself.

Dosage: Take one 1,000 mg. tablet with food at breakfast then at supper time.

Aromatherapy

Basically, there are four ways to use the aromatherapy essential oils from plants: oral, external, nasal (inhalation) and in cooking. Aromatherapy uses the essential oils that are distilled from a whole plant or a specific part of the plant. They are powerful substances that can affect your health and wellbeing.

An essential oil can contain as many as 200 organic chemicals and the combination determines the essential oil's properties. Different essential oils affect different aspects of the body. For example, essential oil of grapefruit is thought to help suppress appetite and stimulate the immune system.

The essential oils are very delicate and volatile. Improper storage or exposure to sun, heat or air and they can easily lose their beneficial properties. With proper storage, a small bottle will last years. A little really goes a long way.

When using essential oils to create aromatherapy massage oils, it is preferable to use 100 percent pure botanical essential oils in them. Synthetic ones may not have the same therapeutic properties. It's not the smell as much as the chemistry of the oils that counts. Read the labels, to see if it is diluted in a carrier base or is 100 percent natural. The more pure the oil, the greater the likelihood it will have therapeutic properties. Smell does not indicate it is 100 percent pure botanical oil.

A stress relieving mixture includes the essential oils of Roman chamomile (3 drops), lavender (4 drops) and orange (3 drops), mixed into a base of 1/4 cup (60 ml) of safflower and 1/4 cup (60 ml) of almond cold-pressed oils. For different emotional states, you can use different oils, in various combinations, with up to 12 drops per half cup of base oils. Experiment with combinations of one or more of the oils to create the synergistic blend that works best for you.

Synergy means the benefit derived from a combination of materials that is greater than the individual components alone. Here's a list of recommended oils for different emotional states:

- **Anxiety:** use basil, bay leaf, lemon balm, orange, sandalwood or ylang-ylang.
- **Depression:** use basil, and for hormonal depression, such as PMS, try clary sage.
- **Tension:** use Canadian pine, lemon balm, rosewood or ylang-ylang.
- **Insomnia:** use tangerine or orange. When you go to sleep, put a drop of orange on your pillow, below your nose and savor the aroma.

Essential oils are prone to rapid deterioration, if stored improperly. This is due to oxidation when exposed to air. In addition, exposure to sunlight, extremes of heat or cold can cause decline in the beneficial properties of an essential oil.

For example, when tea tree oil is exposed to air, it causes the active microbial agent in it, terpinen-4-ol, to decrease. Technically, the Gamma-terpinene content decreases and the para-cymene content increases. Generally, tea tree oil is hardy and does not easily suffer a significant loss of potency when exposed to air, heat or light.

When stored properly, it and other essential oils have a shelf life of approximately three years and have been known to stay potent much longer. Proper storage is important to prevent an essential oil from losing its beneficial properties.

Anxiety: basil, chamomile, jasmine, eucalyptus, marjoram, neroli, ylang-ylang and thyme.

Depression: chamomile, lavender, jasmine, nutmeg and thyme.

Hysteria: chamomile, lavender, jasmine, neroli, nutmeg, rose, peppermint and rosemary.

Irritability: chamomile, cypress, lavender, jasmine,

marjoram, nutmeg, vanilla, Melissa and rose.

Homeopathy

German physician Samuel Hahnemann, founded homeopathy in the early 1800's. There are two different approaches used to create and apply homeopathic remedies. The classical method uses only one single-component remedy at a time. The physician prescribes it in a potency, meaning the number of times the substance is diluted and shaken, specifically adjusted to the patient at that moment in time. Then waits to see what happens before prescribing anything else. Complex homeopathy involves multiple substances, given at the same time, usually in low potencies.

A homeopathic nosode is a super-diluted remedy that takes the energy imprint from a product of disease, such as tuberculosis, bacteria, influenza, measles and about 200 others. No physical traces of the disease are in the nosode. It stimulates the body to rid itself of all "taints" or residues it holds of a disease, whether it was contracted or inherited in a person. Qualified homeopaths are the only ones who administer a nosode.

A homeopathic miasm is the taint or energy residue of a previous illness, even inherited ones across generations. Inherited predispositions for chronic diseases are much more subtle than genetic ones. Broad focused remedies aim at families and people thought to be predisposed to specific illnesses, such as cancer, sexually transmitted diseases, psoriasis and tuberculosis. The remedies are usually available in health food stores, pharmacies and with homeopathic practitioners. How do they work? Primarily by stimulating your body's natural wisdom to heal itself and utilize its self-balancing mechanisms.

The example and remedies listed here are based on personality traits, environmental and other stress inducing situations. The key is to find the remedy that's best suited for you and your particular situation. The better the fit, the greater the chances of successfully using one of these gentle remedies to effectively deal with your stress. Relief can occur within minutes, hours or days. Use one remedy before trying another. Your body takes time to correct the imbalances and problems. Be patient. Potency technically refers to the dilution of the substance. The greater the dilution, the more powerful the homeopathic remedy. In essence, there may not even be one molecule of the actual substance used to energize the water in the solution, yet the solution is more powerful the more times it is diluted and shaken. This is called potentized.

What homeopathic remedies would you use for stress?

Stress indeed is one of the major risk factors that can lead to depression and many other mental disorders. Homeopathy has thousands of formulas. Depending on the nature and traits of the individual and their condition, a course of treatment will be decided on by a homeopathic practitioner, starting with one remedy at a time. Their remedies are significantly more powerful than those you would buy over the counter. The following is a small sampling of remedies for stress related problems. First is the name of the remedy, followed by a dosage range or amount in brackets. The key to successfully using these off the shelf preparations is to choose the one best suited for you and your situation. The closer personality traits and specific situations match the weak spots or underlying tendencies, the greater the chances of the remedy working for you. If you are not sure, consult with a homeopathic practitioner or naturopath, trained in using these remedies.

Colubrina: usually used for stress caused by sleep deprivation or prolonged office work mental work, or studying.

Nat. Mur: relieves symptoms that appear after anger, fright or grief.

Sepia: eases chronic stress or overwork, such as motherhood or pregnancy.

Pulsatilla: for stress, characterized by rapid mood swings, symptoms which wander from place to place or constantly changing physical symptoms.

Sulfur: for a variety of states. This is a deep and broad acting remedy.

Staphysagria: for grief that has been suppressed, anger or indignation.

Natural Vitamins, Minerals and Trace Minerals to help with stress.

Vitamin	Combine with	Source	Therapeutic Applications
B Complex	Vitamins C,E, Calcium, Phosphorus	Brewer's yeast, liver, whole grains	Needed for proper maintenance of the nervous system; proper functioning of the cell and its energy metabolism
B1 (Thiamine)	B complex, Vitamins B2, C, E, Folic Acid, Niacin, Manganese, Sulphur	Brewer's Yeast, Brown Rice, Fish, Meat, Nuts, Organ meats, Poultry, Wheat Germ	Helps maintain good health. Helps maintain normal growth. Helps the body metabolize carbohydrates

B2 (Riboflavin)	B complex, Vitamins B6, C, Niacin, Phosphorus	Nuts, Organ meats, Whole grain	A factor in the maintenance of good health. Helps in tissue formation. Helps the body to metabolize proteins, fats, carbohydrates
B6 (Pyridoxine)	B complex, Vitamins B1, B2, C, Pantothenic Acid Magnesium Potassium Linoleic Acid, Sodium	Brewer's yeast, Green leafy vegetables, Meat, Organ Meats, Wheat Germ Whole grains Desiccated liver	A factor in the maintenance of good health helps the body to metabolize Proteins, Fats, carbohydrates and helps in tissue formation.
B12 (Cobalamin)	B complex, Vitamin B6 C, Choline Inositil Potassium Sodium	Cheese, Fish, Milk, milk products, Organ meats	Helps in treating pernicious anemia. Promotes heart health.
Folic Acid (Folacin B Complex)	B complex Vitamins B12, C, Biotin Pantothenic Acid	Brewer's Yeast, Fish Legumes, Organ meats Soybeans Wheat Germ Lecithin	Adequate intake helps to maintain good health, produce red blood cells and helps prevent neural tube defects when taken prior to becoming pregnant and during early pregnancy
Niacin (Niacinamide	B complex, Vitamins B12,	Brewer's Yeast,	A factor in the maintenance

B Complex)	B2, C, phosphorus	Seafood, Lean meats, Milk, milk products, Poultry, Desiccated liver	of good health. Helps normal growth and development. Helps the body to metabolize proteins, fats, carbohydrates
Pantothenic Acid (B Complex)	B complex, Vitamins B6, B12, C, Biotin, Folic Acid	Brewer's yeast Legumes Organ meats salmon wheat germ, whole grains	A factor in the maintenance of good health, helps the body to metabolize proteins, fats, carbohydrates, and helps in tissue formation
C (Ascorbic Acid)	All vitamins, Minerals BioflvonoidsC alcium Magnesium	Citrus fruits Cantaloupe green peppers	Vitamin C is a factor in the normal development and maintenance of bones, cartilage, teeth and gums. It promotes a healthy immune system and possesses antioxidant activities

Finally...Gems of Wisdom

"Melancholy and other mental ills seem the prerogative of those who are intelligent. You've got to know the world to conclude you can't stand it. Did you ever see a fool that was really depressed?" - Taylor Caldwell, *Testimony of Two Men*

~ ~ ~ ~

"Most people are about as happy as they make up their minds to be." - Abraham Lincoln

~ ~ ~ ~

"Nobody has to stay depressed." - Dr. Harvey Ross

~ ~ ~ ~

"Happiness does not depend on outward conditions. It depends on inner conditions and inner attitudes. It isn't what we have or who we are or where we or what we are doing that makes us happy or unhappy. It is what we think about." - Dale Carnegie

~ ~ ~ ~

"When you wake up, decide to be happy today. Decide it is a beautiful day. Think yourself happy. Be glad for every little thing." - John Haggai

~ ~ ~ ~

"Apathy can be overcome only by enthusiasm. Enthusiasm can be aroused only by two things – an idea which takes your imagination by storm and a definite intelligible plan for carrying that idea into practice." - Arnold Toynbee

"Action seems to follow feeling, but really action and feeling go together; and by regulating the action, which is under the more direct control of the will, we indirectly regulate the feeling which is not. Thus the sovereign voluntary path to cheerfulness, if our cheerfulness be lost, is to sit up cheerfully and to act and speak as if cheerfulness were already there." - Will James

~ ~ ~ ~

Look to this day,

For it is LIFE – the very LIFE of Life

For in its brief course lie all the realities and all the verities of your existence.

The bliss of growth, the glory of action and the splendor of beauty.

For every yesterday is but a dream

And every tomorrow is but a vision

But every today, well lived

Makes every yesterday and dream of beauty

And every tomorrow a vision of hope

Look well, there, to this day.

This is the salutation Life offers to us with each dawn.

REFERENCES

1. Elvis Ali. *The All-In-One Guide to Natural Remedies and Supplements.* Ages Publications, December,1999
2. Cognitive remission: a novel objective for the treatment of major depression?
   Bortolato B, et al.,BMC Med. 2016 Jan 22;14(1):9. doi: 10.1186/s12916-016-0560-3.
3. Can Melatonin Act as an Antioxidant in Hydrogen Peroxide-Induced Oxidative Stress Model in Human Peripheral Blood Mononuclear Cells?
   Emamgholipour S, Hossein-Nezhad A, Ansari M. Biochem Res Int. 2016;2016:5857940. doi: 10.1155/2016/5857940. Epub 2016 Jan 11.
4. Dana Ullman. Homeopathy: Medicine for the 21st Century. North Atlantic Books. 1998
5. Ernst E, White AR. Acupuncture for back pain: a meta-analysis of randomized controlled trials. Arch Intern Med 1998;158:2235-41.
6. Vickers AJ. Can Acupuncture have specific effects on health? A systematic review of acupuncture antiemesis trials. J R Soc Med 1996;89:303-11
7. (2004) Monograph. Withaniasomnifera.Altern Med Rev 9: 211–214.
8. Mishra LC, Singh BB, Dagenais S (2000) Scientific basis for the therapeutic use of Withaniasomnifera(ashwagandha): a review. Altern Med Rev 5: 334–346.
9. Bystritsky A, Kerwin L, Feusner JD. A pilot study of Rhodiolarosea (Rhodax) for generalized anxiety disorder (GAD). J Altern Complement Med 2008;14:175-80
10. L-theanine. Review of Natural Products. Facts &Comparisons Online. April 2010. Accessed April 20, 2016.

11.12. Panossian A, Wagner H. Stimulating effect of adaptogens: an overview with particular reference to their efficacy following single dose administration. PhytotherRes . 2005;19(10):819-838.

12. Kurkin VA, Zapesochnaya GG. Chemical composition and pharmacological properties of Rhodiolarosea .Chem Pharm J . 1986;20(10):1231-1244.

13. Petkov VD, Yaakov D, Mosharoff A, et al. Effects of alcohol aqueous extract from Rhodiolarosea L. roots on learning and memory. ActaPhysiolPharmacolBulg . 1986;12(1):3-16.

14. Saratikov A, Marina TF, Fisanova LL. Effect of golden root extract on processes of serotonin synthesis in CNS. J BiolSci . 1978;6:142.

15. Darbinyan V, Aslanyan G, Amroyan E, Gabrielyan E, Malmstrom C, Panossian A. Clinical trial of Rhodiolarosea L. extract SHR-5 in the treatment of mild to moderate depression. Nord J Psychiatry . 2007;61(5):343-348.

16. Cooley K, et al. (2009) Naturopathic Care for Anxiety: A Randomized Controlled Trial ISRCTN78958974. PLoS ONE 4(8): e6628. doi:10.1371/journal.pone.0006628

17. "American Journal of Clinical Nutrition"; Mechanisms by which botanical lipids affect inflammatory disorders; Chilton FH et al; 2008

18. Cicero AF, Derosa G, Brillante R, et al. Effects of Siberian ginseng (Eleutherococcussenticosus maxim.) on elderly quality of life: a randomized clinical trial. Arch GerontolGeriatrSuppl 2004;9:69-73.

19. Amaryan G, Astvatsatryan V, Gabrielyan E, et al. Double-blind, placebo-controlled, randomized, pilot clinical trial of ImmunoGuard--a standardized fixed

combination of AndrographispaniculataNees, with Eleutherococcussenticosus Maxim, Schizandrachinensis Bail and Glycyrrhizaglabra L. extracts in patients with Familial Mediterranean Fever. Phytomedicine 2003;10:271-85.

20. Kieran, Cooley, et. Al Naturopathic Care for Anxiety: A Randomized Controlled Trial ISRCTN78958974, CCNM. 2009

   a. Natural Health Products Directorate Monograph: Vitamin C. [Internet] [cited March 9th, 2016] Available at: http://www.hc-sc.gc.ca/dhp-mps/prodnatur/applications/licen-prod/monograph/mono_vitamin_c_e.html

23. Natural Health Products Directorate Monograph: Multi vitamins. [Internet] [cited March 9th, 2016] Available at: http://www.hc-sc.gc.ca/dhp-mps/prodnatur/applications/licen-prod/monograph/multi_vitmin_suppl-eng.php

24. Michael Irwin, KavitaVedhara (2005). *Human Psychoneuroimmunology*. Oxford University Press.

25. Rahe RH, Arthur RJ (1978). *"Life change and illness studies: past history and future directions"*. J Human Stress. 4 (1): 3–15.

26. Holmes TH, Rahe RH (1967). *"The Social Readjustment Rating Scale"*. J Psychosom Res. 11 (2): 213–8.

ABOUT THE AUTHOR

Dr. Elvis Ali is highly respected for his work in Naturopathic Medicine. Dr. Elvis, as he is affectionately known, has been in private practice for over 30 years, specializing in Chinese and sports medicine and nutrition. With impressive credentials - Bachelor of Science, majoring in Biology, Licensed Acupuncturist, Doctorate in Naturopathic Medicine; Mind/Body Medicine at Harvard Medical School, Diploma in Homeopathic Medicine - he lectures internationally, has written several books and appeared on radio and television shows. His passion lies in empowering people by educating them on complementary health and wellness, and non-intrusive options.

www.ingramcontent.com/pod-product-compliance
Lightning Source LLC
Chambersburg PA
CBHW070201290526
45789CB00002B/861